YOU'RE DOING GREAT!

YOU'RE DOING GREAT!
AND OTHER LIES ALCOHOL TOLD ME

DUSTIN DUNBAR

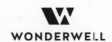

WONDERWELL

Library of Congress Control Number: 2023914916

ISBN 978-1-63756-031-0 (hardcover)
ISBN 978-1-63756-032-7 (EPUB)

Editor: Allison Serrell
Cover design and interior design: Adrian Morgan
Cover image: Shutterstock

Published by Wonderwell in Los Angeles, CA
www.wonderwell.press

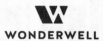

Printed and bound in Canada

To my dearest mother:

Thank you for being the guiding light that leads us toward healing and for showing us the true meaning of love. This book is dedicated to you, with all my love and gratitude.

TABLE OF CONTENTS

INTRODUCTION

Hello. My name is Dustin.

I grew up poor in the Midwest, but I went on to become a model with a doctoral degree in psychology. I retired early by investing in income properties around the United States, and once upon a time, Ryan Seacrest handpicked me to be the "LA Shrink." I have lived all over the world in some of the most beautiful and exotic places there are. Oh, and I married a gorgeous and intelligent woman, and she and I have two beautiful, smart daughters.

I'm not telling you all of this to brag. I'm telling you this to warn you. Despite appreciating everything I had, I almost threw all of it—and so much more—away.

After years of moderate social drinking, I became addicted to alcohol. The irony is that I knew better. I knew exactly the kind of damage and violence that comes from alcohol addiction. Throughout my childhood, I watched my father become addicted to alcohol and abuse my mother verbally and physically. I swore I would never be like him. And yet, I still became addicted to alcohol and ended up behaving exactly like him—maybe even worse.

Before now, I have never told anyone this story. But it's time, and it starts like this.

My ex-wife and I were in Hawaii. We were drinking ice-cold IPAs at a local happy hour and watching Monday Night Football, the exact same thing many Americans do every week during the NFL season. Once the game ended, we continued drinking. Because why not? It's what we always did, and we were having fun. Later, at home, we both had about three glasses of red wine before capping off our night with a cocktail of whiskey over ice. Granted, this was more than we usually drank, but not by much, honestly.

What I recall, which isn't much, is that my ex-wife and I started arguing about something. Neither of us remembers what the fight was about. What we do remember is that we were getting louder and louder, more and more aggressive, until I thought we were going to wake up our daughters.

I can still vaguely see my ex-wife getting right in my face, screaming at the top of her lungs. I remember putting my right hand over her mouth to keep her quiet. I put my left hand behind her neck. I remember tackling her to the bed and her getting up and running out of the room. After a few minutes, I passed out on the bed. I woke up to three police officers, guns drawn, ready to take me to jail.

That is my version of the story—at least, what I recollect.

My ex-wife, however, remembered a much different story. She said that I grabbed her by the throat. She said I picked her up off the floor and started to choke her. She told me she thought she was going to die. She said I threw her on the bed, before she was finally able to run out of the room, gasping for air. Terrified, she grabbed our daughters and fled the house. Once she felt safe, she called the police, who found me passed out on the bed.

Which story is the truth? Mine or hers? I had no idea. All I knew, in my alcohol-deadened mind, was that I was angry. Not at myself. I was still in denial and far too wrapped up in my own ego to imagine I could ever be fully responsible for anything. I was angry at my ex-wife. Sitting in the back of the police car with my hands zip-tied behind my back, I couldn't figure out what I had done that was so bad. I hadn't hit her or choked her. It wasn't even close to as bad as what I had seen my dad do to my mom. I clearly remember thinking this, even with my face smushed against the plexiglass partition of the police car.

I was completely wrong, of course. My addicted, in-denial mind was working overtime. When the police booked me, they showed me photos of my ex-wife. Violent red marks covered her neck. I had done that, I finally understood. I could have killed my ex-wife, the mother of my children. And, just as quickly, I realized I was now *worse* than my dad, a much more dangerous monster.

You're probably thinking this is when I started to turn things around. Surely, you must be thinking this was my rock bottom, that I had finally realized I needed to stop being in denial and start addressing my out-of-control addiction. Alas, dear reader, you have too much faith in me. I was far from done.

I stayed mad at my ex-wife for a month.

"How could she do such a thing?" yelled my fragile, addicted ego. "I am a loving husband and doting father to her children! You were drunk, too, and you wouldn't stop screaming."

I knew I was out of control, but I still couldn't stop drinking. I kept drinking for another year.

I finally hit bottom after drinking heavily on another trip, this time to Canada. My ex-wife and I went on a whiskey-drinking tour with friends. I really didn't want to go. I was already getting tired of drinking. In fact, I went an entire month without drinking before the trip, which made me feel really good. But I agreed to go. It was a disaster. I was blacking out and hitting on women in front of my ex-wife. I was so disrespectful and so careless. At the end of the trip, she told me she was done with me. I knew she meant it. On the flight home, I had a Bloody Mary, which is the last drink of alcohol I ever had.

That was nearly four years ago.

As I write this, we are getting a divorce. She hasn't told me she loves me since that trip, which I understand. Throughout ten years of marriage, all she did was love me, take great care of our children, and make us tons of money; in turn, because of my alcohol addiction and what I later learned was an unconscious love addiction, all I did was traumatize her by sneaking around behind her back until she finally had enough of me and my crap. Today, I live alone in San Diego and, though I share joint custody of our girls, now ages eight and ten, I see in them the same signs of anxiety and stress I experienced as a scared little boy in my father's house.

No person in their "right" mind would do what I did.

THE ALCOHOL MATRIX

But here's the thing: I wasn't in my right mind; I was hardly conscious. I was addicted and I was unconscious. I was blind to my terrible behavior and my crippling dependency. I was in the full grasp of the ugly, insidious, and life-destroying lies alcohol and alcohol culture tell us about drinking. I was caught in what I call the Alcohol Matrix, the collective illusion deep within us that encourages us to drink, more and more, no matter what.

When I finally had my awakening after many years of drinking, I had a lucid dream about alcohol. I was on a hard hospital gurney with alcohol being pumped into me through multiple tubes. As far as my eye could see, there was an endless number of people in the same condition as me, hooked up to the tubes of alcohol, except my eyes were open and the other people were still asleep. Everyone else was alone, but I was surrounded by a motley crew of Alcohol Matrix marketeers: George Clooney in a tux, looking dapper as ever with a shot of Casamigos tequila in hand; the Guinness toucan raising a pint to my health; a French sommelier presenting a bottle of Bordeaux; two bikini-clad girls sipping Coors Lights; and the three Budweiser frogs croaking, "Bud!" "Weis!" "Er!" Beyond them stood a couple of Big Alcohol marketing executives in suits.

As I squirmed in fear and rage, trying to get the tubes out of me, I could hear them talking to one another. George looked down at me and said, "It looks like he is waking up."

The others chimed in.

"Don't let him!"

"Give him more!"

"Dustin, you can't live a fun, sexy life without it."

"It is good for you."

"Just put the tubes back in. It will take the edge off."

"No one else is going to live alcohol-free with you."

I stood up on the gurney, and I ripped the tubes out of me. "Get the hell away from me!" I shouted. I woke up in a sweat, but finally fully awake.

The concept of the Alcohol Matrix came to me from that dream.

A month after the dream, I was reading a book titled *The Unexpected Joy of Being Sober* by Catherine Gray. She says, "There's a jaw-dropping scene in the film *The Matrix*, which sums up, for me, how it feels to unplug from our alcohol-centric society. It's a swooping sci-fi shot which shows an endless field of people plugged into a fake reality." I was beyond shocked that she and I had the same revelation. And that is when I realized that since she was in England and I was in California, it was a collective experience.

Long before any of us were even alive, the Alcohol Matrix was spinning its lies. And, as a child, years before you took your first sip of alcohol, you were already being conditioned to believe them. Throughout human history, alcohol has been our most accessible painkiller. It has also been consumed in celebration for every major life event in nearly every culture, from parties and weddings to religious rituals and funerals. And, thanks to the Alcohol Matrix, we've all been brainwashed to believe alcohol (literal ethanol) is totally safe to consume, and rather than getting us sick or ruining our lives, alcohol is actually good for us. You and I have been brainwashed to believe alcohol is the secret to being cool, attractive, fun, and carefree.

I knew better. And *you* knew better. But you and I continued to drink, primarily because of our collective belief that alcohol benefits us in some way, even though we were fully aware of the damage alcohol does to our personal and professional lives, and study after study that proves alcohol causes cancer and *two hundred* other diseases.[1]

Every time you raise a glass of alcohol to your lips, there is a part of you, deep down, that knows you're doing something unhealthy, stupid, and self-destructive. It might just be a tiny voice in the back of your head. But it's there, nagging at you. That little voice is you waking up from the Alcohol Matrix. You are starting to see how profound it is. Once you see it fully, you'll realize it's an absolute monster, and it is everywhere. It's influencing you unconsciously, telling you how to behave and what's expected of you. Get together with loved ones, and the Alcohol Matrix sets unspoken rules. Host or attend a social gathering, and the Alcohol Matrix shapes your actions in numerous ways. It is an ancient, unconscious, powerful social signal that you tune into without question.

Think about how many times you've either said or heard

someone say the following:

"You deserve a drink to take the edge off."

"Just one won't hurt."

"It's beer o'clock."

You know deep down that alcohol is bad for you. Science has proven it is bad for you. Unfortunately, you've continued to drink it because you've continued to believe these and other lies the Alcohol Matrix tells you, just like I did.

"Drink me, your life will have less pain."

"Drink me, you will have more friends, more money, a better party, more sex, a nicer car, better body, more laughs; you will look cool, sophisticated, and classy."

"Drink me, you will be funnier."

"Drink me, people will like you more."

It goes on and on and on.

You know exactly what I'm talking about. You can feel it, just like I did. You might not be able to explain it, but you can sense a dark side to the emphasis everyone seems to place on drinking. Maybe you've always noticed it, or perhaps you just started to see it recently. Maybe you're finally starting to notice how things could—and *should*—actually be. Right now, this creeping realization might still just be a tiny voice in the back of your head. Listen to that voice because it's telling you the truth. It's trying to show you what's real. It's trying to remind you about who you truly are. It took me far too long to listen to this voice, and because I failed to heed its warning, I hurt everyone I loved and nearly threw away everything I valued most. After suffering through an unbelievable (and unbelievably long) amount of pain, I finally started to listen to this voice, which kicked off a remarkable process of personal transformation and a radical shift in consciousness.

The truth is, alcohol is addictive. Anyone—and I mean

anyone—who consumes enough of it will become addicted to it, just as anyone would taking any other addictive substance, whether it's tobacco or heroin, Vicodin or OxyContin. Some people get hooked faster than others. Maybe you were introduced to alcohol early in life, when addiction susceptibility peaks. Maybe you were born into a heavy-drinking family, like I was, in which addiction is practically protocol. Maybe you are like the 70 percent of heavy drinkers who experienced childhood trauma and, to alleviate the pain, self-medicate with alcohol. Regardless, *anyone* has the potential to become addicted to alcohol once they consume enough of it.

Just like me.

Here are some more truths:

You are not the problem; alcohol is.
You are not allergic to alcohol.
You don't have an addictive personality.
You don't have the alcoholic's gene.
You are not defective.
You don't need to drink.

I know this is probably hard to believe, but it's the truth. And it's time you accept it.

Don't make the same mistake that I did and think that if you get all the external things you dreamed of in your life, they will give you peace. External things and accomplishments come and go. What has made me truly peaceful and joyous is to be completely cured of alcohol addiction and finally free of the Alcohol Matrix of lies, which has allowed me to grow spiritually from the inside out and begin the process of healing the broken parts of myself that in turn broke apart my life.

I have been alcohol-free for the four years it has taken me to write this book. I am not sober. Sober means somber, subdued, serious, solemn, grave, and restrained. I am none of those things. Nor am I an alcoholic. I am a joyous, alcohol-free man.

In the *The Art of War*, Sun Tzu's advice is to know your enemy, and man, did I come to know my enemy. Over the past four years, I have read, researched, and studied some of the brightest experts and theories on addiction. I have pored over every study and every cultural account of alcohol I could find to figure out why and how it became the elixir of adult life, a constant at every party and every important milestone. I have read and reread books about addiction and recovery that resonated most with me. I have repeated statistics and facts about alcohol over and over as if they were my personal mantra. I also had a lot of therapy . . . a *lot* of therapy. Besides weekly sessions, I attend a love addiction program based on the 12-step program of Alcoholics Anonymous (AA), which is ironic because AA didn't help me at all for my alcohol addiction. (Believe me, I'll have more on this later.)

Slowly but surely I've removed the chains of my alcohol addiction, and my fear of abandonment is now healed. I am living my life peacefully on my own terms, without the need to grasp for any external substance or any readily available person in a futile attempt to make myself feel better or loved. I am grateful and present. Being present also means recognizing how many other men are not.

Look, I love being a guy, and on my best days, I like to consider myself a guy's guy. But after reading some truly troubling statistics, I had to start facing some equally disturbing questions about the relationship between alcohol and masculinity:

- Almost 58 percent of adult men report drinking alcohol in the past 30 days compared with 49 percent of adult women, according to the Centers for Disease Control and Prevention (CDC).[2]

- Men are also more likely to binge drink than women—21 percent compared with 13 percent.[3]

- Among men who binge drink, one in four drink to excess at least five times a month and, on average, consume at least nine drinks during a drinking session.[4]

- In 2020, the most recent available data point, 13 percent of men said they had an alcohol use disorder compared with 9 percent of women.[5]

- On average, men not only drink more than women, but we also have a harder time "dealing" with alcohol. We are hospitalized more often with alcohol-related incidents than women. Approximately 97,000 men die every year in the United States as a result of excessive drinking.[6]

- Binge drinking increases aggression, which increases the risk of physical assault and sexual violence.

- Men are also more than three times as likely to die by suicide than females, and more likely to have been drinking prior to suicide.[7]

Learning statistics like these is one of the reasons I decided to write this book. In addition to telling you the truth about alcohol, I'm also going to lay down some uncomfortable facts about men and drinking, and specifically about an aspect of masculinity that too often encourages the kinds of destructive behavior I just listed. Although I have no doubt this book will also speak to women struggling with alcohol, men have sadly been overlooked in this category. Most of the popular titles about recovery and living alcohol-free are written by women for women, which is great. But this is primarily a book for men by a man. In the following pages, I'm going to expose the lies men all too willingly accept about alcohol, from "You're Not Really a Man if You Don't Drink" and "One Drink Won't Kill You" to "Alcohol

Washes Away the Pain" and "You're the Problem, Not Alcohol."

The goal of this book is threefold: to disabuse you of the culturally constructed delusion that alcohol has any benefit whatsoever, to make you aware of the truth about alcohol, and to make you see that you are not defective. In each chapter, I will detail and then debunk eleven lies I personally believed about alcohol. There are others, obviously, but I believe these eleven lies are the most pernicious. At the very least, these eleven lies affected me most of all. Some chapters might speak more directly to your own experiences with alcohol than others. That's totally okay! Everyone's relationship with alcohol is different. If a chapter title resonates more with you than another, that's great. Start with that one. I wrote this book to educate and empower people who want to become alcohol-free. I also wrote it to entertain people. Though the chapters are laid out in a loose chronology of my life, you don't have to read them from start to finish to get something out of the book. The details of my biography aren't really what this book is about. It's really about the lessons I learned when I finally started to interrogate the lies I all too readily accepted about alcohol while I was trapped in the Alcohol Matrix.

Regardless of how you decide to read the book, I am fully confident that the lessons I share will help you start to interrogate the many other ways alcohol lied to you in the past and continues to lie to you today. My hope is that my stories, no matter how embarrassing or damning they prove to my own character, will not only make you aware of these lies but also help you accept the truth about alcohol and, in the process, start living your life peacefully on your own terms: alcohol-free and fully awake.

To guide you during your journey, I include a Detox Timeline, which describes what I felt during my own transformation from a life of drinking to an alcohol-free existence. I offer some insight about this experience from the first week to two years being alcohol-free. Again, I write about my own experiences. Your perspective and experiences may be different. The Detox Timeline is there to encourage you in your journey, not to determine it. Think of it as a reference point, not a road map. There are many roads you can take to become alcohol-free—as many roads as there are to Rome.

THIS NAKED MIND

The irony is that it took an advertising executive with no background in mental health or medicine named Annie Grace to cure me of my alcohol addiction. Her book *This Naked Mind* woke me from my unconscious "alcohol benefits me" illusion and completely cured me of my cravings for alcohol. This book follows in Annie's footsteps. She did the hard labor with her extensive research and professional resources, and I will happily take the quick road and refer to her impeccable work. She does a wonderful job of reprogramming the individual unconscious mind's erroneous beliefs about alcohol. By addressing the collective unconscious with clear eyes, this book takes it a step further, exposing the lies alcohol continues to tell us and the lies we continue to tell ourselves about alcohol. Annie Grace says to pay it forward and "be brave and vulnerable, letting those who still suffer know they are not alone in their struggle."

This is the second reason I wrote this book: to pay it forward.

This effort is the genesis of The Alcohol-Free Revolution (AFR; www.WeAretheAFR.org), a nonprofit group coaching program I launched that brings people from all around the world together and supports them in their journey to becoming alcohol-free. The hour-long Zoom sessions are free for anyone to join, although a donation of ten dollars is recommended. These sessions are called 100 percent U. The U is for university and, of course, you. We stole . . . I mean . . . we borrowed our slogan from Liverpool, my favorite soccer team . . . I mean . . . football club: *You'll never walk alone*. Right now, it's a community, but it will soon be a movement.

The final reason I wrote this book is my daughters, Tallulah and Milly. Four years ago, I was contemplating what Annie said about paying it forward and writing my story. I came across a quote on my phone that said, "One day you will tell your story of how you overcame your addiction to alcohol, and it will become someone else's survival guide." I wrote that quote on a piece of scrap paper on my desk. The next day, I looked at the paper, and underneath my handwriting was a note from my six-year-old daughter that read, "whoevr rote this tank you I love u." It was the first note she ever wrote me. "Ahh crap," I said to myself. "Now I have to write a book."

So, although I hope you benefit from this book, if all it ever does is help my two daughters see through our culture's illusions and misinformation about alcohol, then it will still be a complete success for me.

My goal is also to keep the book fun. Sometimes we make life out to be way more serious than it really is, and I am positive that we can all have a laugh while we change. Even as children, most of us were helplessly addicted to the hokey pokey, but we turned ourselves around. (Yikes! I will try to do better with my jokes.)

One more thing before we dive in: if you identify as an alcoholic, this book probably isn't for you. I don't believe in alcoholics. I believe people can get addicted to alcohol and, just like a two-packs-a-day smoker who gave up cigarettes because they realized they were disgusting cancer sticks, people who are actively addicted to alcohol can quit drinking and be disgusted by alcohol and have zero desire to drink cancer juice.

A friend of mine recently asked what I thought about his drinking. I already knew how much he had consumed in his life, for how long, and how often. I told him that because of how much he had consumed, he was most likely addicted to alcohol.

He got very nervous and defensive, and asked in a hushed voice, "You really think I am an alcoholic?"

"Absolutely not." I replied. "I think you are addicted to alcohol."

His defensiveness was gone. He was now curious about this statement. "What's the difference?" he asked.

"The difference is that with an alcoholic, the person is seen as the issue. When a person is addicted to alcohol, the substance is the issue."

This perspective is key to exposing the Alcohol Matrix.

Sorry, one more thing before we begin. Becoming alcohol-free is not a competition. There are as many ways to become alcohol-free as there are people addicted to alcohol. You and your path are unique, and you will become alcohol-free in your own way. This book is simply the story of how I was able to become completely cured of all cravings for alcohol. Although I hope to inspire you, if you find a way that feels better to you, please follow that path. If anyone tells you their way is the only way . . . run, don't walk, away from them.

All my love,
Dustin

DETOX TIMELINE: ONE WEEK ALCOHOL-FREE

You can do this. Trust me.

I became alcohol-free in Hawaii, on September 19, 2019. The Bloody Mary I had on my flight back from that disaster of a trip to Canada is the last drop of alcohol I've had since. When I ordered it, I knew it was my last drink.

Most of you won't need to take a final drink. You might already be done with—and disgusted by—alcohol. But for those of you who need to take your last drink, do it. Don't beat yourself up. You're saying a final goodbye to something that was in your life for a long time. That part of your life is now in the past.

Just know that it is an absolute fact that you're putting a toxic poison into your body. Mentally, it is important to get your consciousness in order, with no illusion about alcohol's benefits. You have to know with every fiber of your being that alcohol is bad for you, in every possible way.

The most important thing in this first seven days is community. Having people in your corner is essential. During my first week being alcohol-free, I relied on a community I found on the I Am Sober app. It was the best twelve dollars (a month) I ever spent. People posted regularly about their initial struggles and small but important successes. I spent that first week typing and texting, checking in with my online community, sharing positive reinforcement with people who were going through the same thing I was going through at the same time. We were all walking the same walk, and we were determined to keep each other accountable and make everyone feel supported. I felt like I was part of a team. (Now you, too, can be a teammate at the AFR website: www.WeAretheAFR.org)

When I wasn't on the app, I was hyperfocused on researching

alcohol, which I realize now was the first step in unbrainwash-
ing my mind. Almost immediately, I realized how bad alcohol
is, how destructive and pernicious it is. Did you know alcohol is
just ethanol, a highly flammable organic compound that is also
used in personal care products, paints and varnishes, and gasoline? A liquid toxin, ethanol is the active ingredient in every
alcoholic drink you've ever swallowed.

At the same time, I realized the power of repetition as reinforcement. I read and reread the books that resonated with me
most. I repeated statistics and facts about alcohol, again and
again, as if they were my personal mantra. You can do the same,
especially if and when intrusive thoughts and temptations arise:
keep reminding yourself of the facts about alcohol and the harm
it can cause.

I was on a mission. Not only to break my addiction, but to
break out of the Alcohol Matrix and its network of insidious lies
once and for all.

My other allies in this mission were exercise and meditation,
which helped me get my body and mind right after years of
beating them up. Take a brisk walk, practice yoga, take fitness
classes, ride a bike, or play with your kids. Meditation helps quiet
your mind, training it on your own thoughts rather than the lies
you've accepted about drinking and about yourself all these years.
The guided meditation app Headspace is my personal favorite. It
costs about six dollars a month, which is how much I used to
spend for one drink! Now I spend that same amount to listen to a
fully ordained Buddhist monk from London named Andy guide
me through my meditation and explain in understandable ways
what is happening in my brain to influence my thoughts. Get the
app, do the daily guided meditation for ten to twenty minutes,
and before you know it you will be a "meditator" just like me.
Exercise and meditation will help you as your body starts to rid

itself of all those horrible toxins.

WITHDRAWAL SYMPTOMS

My addiction looked like two glasses of wine per night and more on the weekends. I didn't experience a lot of discomfort or withdrawal when I went alcohol-free, but it is very normal for your body and your mind to feel not so great when you are overcoming physical and psychological addiction while also purging your system of a lot of toxins. Depending on your level of addiction and the quantity of alcohol you regularly consume, detoxing might initially cause you some discomfort—mild, moderate, or severe. It's possible, if not probable, that you may experience a racing heartbeat, "the sweats," "the shakes," panic, or sudden mood swings. Though scary, withdrawal symptoms, no matter how debilitating, are only temporary.

If you are more severely addicted or have serious cravings, consult with your doctor. Three types of oral medications (naltrexone, acamprosate, and disulfiram) are currently approved for treating alcohol addiction. All three can mitigate symptoms of withdrawal, and all three can make alcohol undesirable to drink. Naltrexone, for instance, helps reduce cravings by binding and blocking the opioid receptors in the brain, which blocks alcohol's sedative effects. Acamprosate interacts with the brain's neurotransmitter systems, which reduces the addictive effects of alcohol, and disulfiram causes an adverse reaction to alcohol, like vomiting, nausea, a throbbing headache, and dizziness.

Symptoms of withdrawal can also be intensified by poor overall health. Those of you who don't eat a nutritious diet or get regular exercise will experience more unpleasant withdrawal symptoms. This is because your bodies are less resilient. Likewise, if you smoke, use other drugs, or have health conditions like depression, chronic pain, or underperforming organs, you might have some negative symptoms when going alcohol-free.

If you suffer from these or other diagnosed conditions, I suggest you talk with a doctor to help you start to detox from alcohol.

Remember—you sacrifice nothing by giving up alcohol. Without it, you gain everything.

PART I

ME, MYSELF, AND I (AND A FEW OTHER PEOPLE)

CHAPTER 1

The Lie Alcohol Told Me:
"You're Not Really a Man If You Don't Drink"

The Truth I Figured Out:
I Don't Have to Prove My Worth

You've probably seen this scene before: a cowboy is puffing on a cigarillo at the long bar of a Western saloon when the villain bursts through the swaying double doors.

"I got a bone to pick with you, pardner!"

The hero ashes his smoke and nods at the bartender. "Hit me," he says smoothly, and a shot of whiskey slides across the wooden counter into the cowboy's hand.

The bartender speaks up. "Why don't you fellas take this outside? I got a business to run here!"

The villain huffs and heads outside. The hero knocks back the whiskey, winks at the girl serving drinks, then makes sure his revolver is loaded.

Outside, the hero and the villain face off. Every townsperson, from the lady to the stable hand, is watching. No one dares take a breath.

"Draw!" The hero whips out his revolver and *boom!* A bullet strikes the villain right between the eyes! The town rejoices, and the hero heads back to the bar without even looking back. The girls swarm him, and he buys a round for the whole place.

Growing up in the Midwest in the 1980s, the decade of Hulk Hogan, Rambo, and Ronald Reagan, that's what I thought being a man was all about. Popular culture, particularly Western movies, taught me to associate alcohol with manhood, even while I saw it turning my father into a domestic abuser. From a young age, I was inundated with red-blooded country ideology. See exhibit A, which is a photo of me at age fourteen with my siblings and my dad.

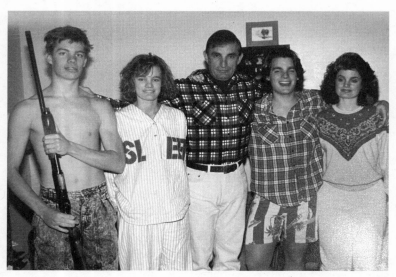

Memories from the Wild West of adolescence!

What can I say? Puberty was rough! I would like to take a brief moment to say I am a game bird–hunting gun owner who is against automatic rifles for public use. If I could save one adult or student from a mass shooting, I would happily give up my bird-hunting shotgun as well. Bow hunting is the best way to hunt anyway, including game birds. But, if any o' you fellers out there comes a-courtin' my girls, me 'n' ol' Bessy will be a-waitin' fer ya!

The midwestern credo of American manhood says a guy like me should be able to take down a double shot of bourbon without flinching. You should love the burn and, as soon as you swallow it down, order another round. This culture told me that you have to drink to be a man—and not only drink, but knock back whiskey like it's your god-given right.

Well, this same god-given right also cost me and my family plenty.

Two generations before I was even a glimmer in my parents' eyes, my great-grandfather struck it rich during the Oklahoma land rush, securing through some pluck and some luck some of the best property in the country. He was an original Sooner of state lore, a local legend who seemed to have secured a fortune for himself and his family that would trickle down to his great-grandchildren. That was the plan, anyway. My great-grandfather drank it all away: every last parcel of land and every penny in his pocket. He never recovered, financially or emotionally, and his tragic story was constantly whispered about in our family as a cautionary tale on the dangers of alcohol. But that didn't stop a lot of us from drinking.

My grandfather, his son, was infamous for his whiskey bingers, which often lasted two weeks. To come down from his binge, he would settle in with a twelve-pack of beer, just to reenter civilized society and stay in the same house as his family.

What's that Bruce Springsteen line about a father wishing that his kids' mistakes would be their own? If I can't remember it now, I don't imagine my grandfather, who never heard of the Boss, was too concerned about passing on his wrongdoings to his son.

Throughout my childhood, I witnessed my father drinking beer to "unwind after a long day." One beer after work quickly became three or four, and he would then turn to a bottle of vodka. Ironically, he didn't drink much until he was around twenty-five years old, not too long before he settled down with my mother and started his own family. Rather than a lifelong project, his addiction was a quick descent.

Let's just say my father was a complicated man, a character who could light up a room or destroy it, depending on his mood or how much liquor was in him. He had a great sense of humor, a keen intellect, and devilish good looks. He was a college professor and basketball coach, an intellectual and athletic powerhouse. He knew it, and he wanted everyone else to know it, too. Whereas other parents were fine with picking their kids up from school or the local pool in wood-bodied station wagons and chaste family sedans, my father, in full peacock mode, preferred to pull up conspicuously in his brown Trans Am, a golden eagle emblazoned across the hood, wearing sunglasses and a brown felt cowboy hat plumed with an arch of feathers. Sometimes, he asked my mother to drop him off a couple of miles from the house so he could jog home, showing off his toned legs, which were exposed thanks to his then very much in style Sansabelt shorts, the kind high school baseball and football coaches made popular long before Irish actor Paul Mescal revitalized 5-inch inseam shorts. My father thought he was Burt Reynolds in *Smokey and the Bandit*, and the ladies ate it up.

My brother, Darron, who'll you'll learn more about over the course of this book, once taught acting classes at a senior center in Oklahoma City. One of his students, who was well into her seventies, approached him after class.

"Are you related to Fred Dunbar?" she asked.

Darron told her he was his son.

"Oh Lord! I could have been your stepmother! He taught me back when I was in college, and all the girls were crazy for him!"

She looked off dreamily, reminiscing about her salad days.

"Mmmmm, I remember he used to wear black underwear with white pants."

Darren told me that story more than a year ago, and I am still not fully uncringed.

These are the things we can laugh at. But take that same Burt Reynolds wannabe and put some vodka in him, and believe me, there's nothing to laugh at. Once my father let the spirit out of that bottle, that spirit sure seemed to take over. I remember sitting in the car in the driveway with my three older siblings. I was probably five years old. I watched my dad turn into a complete alcohol-induced monster. He was yelling, and he dragged my mom out of the house by her hair. She was screaming, begging him to stop. After he threw my mom into the driver's seat, he looked through the car window at me and my siblings—his four children—sitting in the backseat. I could see in his eyes that he was no longer there. Alcohol hadn't taken the edge off; it had taken him over completely.

Another time, after their divorce, my mom was going out. Her date was sitting on our couch, watching TV, and enjoying a cold glass of iced tea. Suddenly, out of nowhere, my father came pounding through the front door, full of rage. With his cowboy-booted leg, he kicked the living room table, sending the man's iced tea all the way up to the ceiling.

Unbeknownst to us, he had already keyed the entire side of the man's car. My dad was yelling at the man, threatening him. But mom's date remained perfectly calm. He just sat there and stared at the television, content to ignore the huge raging man in front him, who was desperate and in need of a reason to throw the first punch. My mom's night was ruined—and her life was likely ruined, too. Her life and her children's lives were all affected in a way that just isn't measurable by their physical health. The damage that alcohol does to the individual drinker is horrible.

The damage that alcohol does to the people around them who have never even taken a drink will affect them in a million indescribable ways for years to come.

And yet, despite swearing I would never go anywhere near alcohol before I was tall enough to ride the bumper cars at the county fair, I still drank, thinking I wouldn't end up like all the other men in my family, who also probably thought they didn't have a problem. Like them, I initially drank to fit in. Later, I drank to prove my own worth as a man. Both reasons, I finally figured out, stem from the same root problem.

WOULDN'T YOU LIKE TO BE A PEPPER, TOO?

The first time I got drunk, I was a sophomore in high school. I was at a pool party with guys from the basketball team. I was drinking a Dr Pepper and having a great time until the girl I'd been crushing on all year showed up. I suddenly had a hard time breathing. I'd seen and thought about this girl almost every day at school, but I didn't have many chances to talk with her because we had different classes. When I did run into her, I was always too chicken to strike up a conversation. With a flat-top haircut, huge metal braces protruding from my mouth, and a beautiful bouquet of red acne all over my face, I wasn't exactly a catch. My confidence was a little low, especially with girls. But at this pool party, I couldn't help but recognize that this might be my chance. My crush was standing right in front of me, looking gorgeous in her red bikini.

My friend, the six-foot-four defensive end from the football team, came up and put his hand on my back. He knew I was into this girl and could tell I was debating talking to her.

"Dustin," he whispered in my ear, "you can do this; go talk to her."

I opened my mouth, but words wouldn't come out. It felt like my chest was being squeezed in a vise. My pulse raced in my ears, and my vision narrowed. *I can't do this*, I thought. *I need help. What will I say? I am an athlete, not a smooth talker. What if there is just an awkward silence? Or what if she laughs at me?*

"Relax," my friend said. "This'll help."

He slid a beer can sideways into my hand. He had poked a large hole in the bottom with a key. "Open your throat, put your mouth on the hole, then tip it up and open the can." I took a deep breath and did it. The cold beer rushed down my throat. It burned like hell.

A few seconds later, I introduced myself to the girls, and we chatted. I had another beer with them and started to feel like I was part of the "in crowd."

I went home that night extremely conflicted. I was furious for slipping up on my promise to not drink alcohol. But I was also elated about connecting with the girl of my dreams. I started rationalizing. *Maybe I can handle my alcohol*, I thought. *How will I know for sure unless I try for myself, right?*

Soon enough, my acne cleared up, the braces came off, I got a decent haircut, and that girl became my high school sweetheart. And it turned out that she liked me as a person, not because I drank beer. But by then I had been conditioned to believe that alcohol was the only way I could fit in, the only way to get what I truly wanted. That was really the first lie alcohol told me, and the first one I believed.

The second lie was that I needed to drink to be a man, which was just as insidious, but probably more destructive because I spent too many years trying to prove to myself—and to others— that I was a man. A man's man, a Western-like hero who's always composed and always in control. The truth was, however, that I was almost never in control, especially when I was drinking. It took me too long to realize this. Like falling into bankruptcy, my capitulation to this lie happened slowly, then all at once. And it started innocuously enough, even if, in retrospect, I can now see the warning signs, which were as subtle as a missing tooth. Let me explain.

By the age of twenty, I had rarely visited anywhere outside of Oklahoma, let alone outside the United States. When I was in college, I had a chance to be an exchange student at West Lancashire College, just outside of Liverpool. I was totally out of place and lost. This was before cell phones and GPS. I think it took me longer to get from the London airport to Liverpool than it did from Oklahoma City to London.

My second day there, I went to the school's bar, where all the faculty and students were having a get-together for the beginning of the school year. I stood there among the crowd feeling very alone and out of place, insecurely drinking my third pint of ale. Finally, a female student spoke to me, and after we chatted about the area for a while, she asked me to sit down in a private booth with her. A few minutes later, a drunk male student came out of nowhere and flopped down basically on top of her and spilled most of his beer on her. Visibly annoyed, she gathered herself and politely introduced him as her friend from her hometown. He looked me over. I could tell he was sizing me up. He put his arm around the girl's shoulders and neck. She squirmed to get loose. I stood up, went to the edge of the table, and told him to let her go.

He stood and put his Liverpool nose directly up to my Okie nose. Then he spit saliva and beer all over my face. "You fookin' American poofta!" and pushed his finger into my left eye.

At the time, I had no idea what a "poofta" was, but I knew it was not a compliment. I now know it's a derogatory slur Neanderthals like this guy too often hurl when they're drunk and looking for a fight. I should have turned my dry other cheek, but

I was twenty years old, still full of anger, and severely jet-lagged, with three strong pints of ale in me. I was having none of it.

I reached back across the Atlantic with my right hand and high-fived the Statue of Liberty, then let my new friend full of ale have a nice "howdy partner" American fist to his left cheek. He went down in a Liverpudlian puddle. His buddy, who was standing behind me, shattered a bottle of beer on the table and put its jagged edge up under my chin. Thankfully, a large bald guy from the crowd pulled the jagged bottle away from my neck and calmed everyone down.

The next day, the same bald guy introduced himself as the captain of the rugby team. Impressed with what he had witnessed the day before, he asked me to join the team. I had played American football and thought rugby would be virtually the same thing (but without pads or a helmet). I was extremely wrong. To the naked eye, rugby and American football may look a lot alike, but the only things they have in common are the field (known as the "pitch"), the goalposts, and the shape of the ball. After that, it is a completely different sport.

WIG OF THE MATCH

I had two quick practices and suddenly found myself on the pitch for the start of a match with a rival university. Just before kickoff, I looked around at the other players, and they had tape circling their heads and mouth guards hanging from their lips. No one had bothered to tell me to tape my head or get a mouth guard. I thought the tape looked funny and didn't have a country-boy clue what it was for. As I looked down at myself in my cleats, socks, shorts, and T-shirt, I analyzed the size of the players on the other team and thought, *This doesn't feel right; even poofta soccer players get to wear shin guards!*

As we engaged the other team's scrum, when each team links

arms and lunges headfirst toward the other team, I felt my left ear rip. It wasn't too painful, as apparently ears don't have a lot of nerves in them, but ears sure can bleed. Blood was everywhere, and my ear was hanging down, almost halfway split from my head. I showed the ref. He blew his whistle and stopped the match to take a look. All he did, though, was smile with his crooked, stained teeth and say, "Jus' a lil' blood, mate. Go on anotha' go."

A player from the other team was upset that I stopped the match to have my ear checked, and of course called me a poofta. At that second, my mind went into fight-or-flight mode. I unfortunately chose fight (which I always seemed to do in my younger, more aggressive drunk days), but I also had a plan to get tossed out of the match. With my cranked-up fight mode and helter-skelter scheme to get the ref to disqualify me, I now viewed this as an all-out, kill-or-be-killed war with the other team. I threw clothesline forearms to their ball carriers' heads. I mashed body parts of every kind with my knees and cleats. I dove on piles of bodies kamikaze-style, with both elbows blared out. I didn't care about the rules, the game, or the score; I just wanted to go get stitches in my hanging ear.

It was pure anarchy until, all of a sudden, I intercepted a pass and ran eighty meters (like yards, but longer) to the left corner of our end zone, whose name I still don't know. I stood there with the ball in my hand, looking back at everyone else, equal parts shocked and triumphant. I was expecting my team and our fans to be rejoicing and happy, but they were all yelling and waving at me to get down. I saw the other team running at me, picking up speed. *What the hell do I need to do?* The fastest member of my team made it to me first and swiped the ball from me just before we both got obliterated by one of the other team's players. The three of us were lying in the end zone (or whatever it's called), and my teammate slammed the ball to the ground. The ref blew the whistle to finally signal a touchdown (or whatever it's called). Face down on that glorious, foggy, cold November day with mud and blood in my eyes, I heard my captain define the situation for the other team, loud enough that many of the fans could hear it as well: "He's American."

Later in the match, my front-right top tooth connected with a Scouser's head and split to the root. (A Scouser is a person from Liverpool. The name fits these compassionate, kind, and sophisticated rugby gentlemen to a tee.) The match ended mercilessly. To this day, my body has never been so completely torn up as it was at that moment. All I wanted was a doctor and a dentist. I asked my captain where I could find both. It didn't matter which one I saw first.

"Nah, mate, not yet," he replied. My compassionate Scouser rugby captain informed me that after the match, the tradition is to go have a drink (or seven) with the other team. *WHAT?* I screamed—but silently, as I did not want to be called a poofta again, especially by my team's captain. *I need serious medical attention!*

At the pub, the other team awarded me "Wig of the Match," or player of the match. I didn't know or care at the time what the wig thing meant, but they lifted me from my muddy chair, put a large blond feminine wig over my mud- and blood-encrusted head, and made me stand on a stage in front of a huge crowd with the other team's Wig of the Match. *Okay, haha, very funny,* I thought as I started to limp my way off the stage.

But no, that was not the end of being Wig of the Match. Now it was time to enjoy a fresh pint, filled half with Guinness and half with whatever else the other team decided to throw in there. As I watched my sworn enemies put mayonnaise, mustard, Tabasco, beans, and salt in my drink, my stomach began to turn.

The other Wig and I had to get the whole disaster pint down while the entire pub of sophisticated Brits sang the light classical tune "Zulu Warrior."

"Get it down! You Zulu warrior!" yelled the entire pub as I gulped and gagged on my eclectic cocktail. "Get it down! You Zulu chief! Chief! Chief!"

I was about halfway done and realized that was the end of the song. The other Wig had his pint of swill all down. This meant I got to have a whole new pint and try to get it down in the approximately eleven seconds it took for the pub to sing the song again. I tried round two with all my might. No luck, and now the whole pub of Scousers was pointing at me at the end of the song while screaming a well-coordinated and compassionate rendition of, "You sad bastard! You sad bastard!"

My sworn enemies took it easy on me for round three, given my pitiful condition. They knew I was not going to be able to choke their spicy pig slop down, so they just left it at a Guinness. I got the regular pint down in the allotted time and immediately ran off the stage to a loo that, thankfully, had no queue, and threw up like I had never heard anyone, man or beast, throw up before. Do you know how bad a front tooth split down to the root hurts when you projectile vomit through it? I hope you never do.

After the pub, I went to the A&E (accident & emergency, or what we Americans call the ER). I looked like the monster Sloth from the movie *The Goonies*. I thought about yelling, "Hey you guys!" in the fun way he always did, but my entire being hurt way too much for any yelling. The doctor looked me up and down, shook his head, and said, "Ah mate, they fooked you up a bit. Well, did you win?"

Looking back on this now, although the rugby scene was easily when I felt the most intense peer pressure to drink alcohol, its lesson is much more insidious. The moral of this story—and the story about the first time I got drunk—is how easy it is to slip into bad habits and bad behavior, and how easy it is to fall prey to all the old, bad clichés of acting like a man. That nervous kid trying to find the courage to talk to his high school crush? That cocky college student who was willing to risk his appendages and intestinal lining to prove he was one of the guys? They're the same guy who, with a beautiful wife and young kids at home, later drunkenly texted his attractive Uber driver for sex on a golf trip with a bunch of other men. They're the same guy who slipped into the back room of a strip club on that same golf trip and then again on another golf trip later. They're the same guy who, shortly after those trips, went to a massage parlor for sex.

Whether I was a sophomore in high school, a college student, or a fully grown man with a wife and kids at home, I continued to believe the lie that, if I didn't drink, I wasn't truly a man, and if I wasn't a man, no one would ever love me. Because I'd watched my father beat my mother, and because he later abandoned me, I unconsciously grasped for attention, validation, and love from alcohol and people my whole life. I became unconsciously addicted to trying to get others to love me. To do that, however, I needed to show the objects of my affection that I was a man worthy of their love—at least, that's what made sense in my warped, alcohol-buzzed state.

CHAPTER 2

The Lie Alcohol Told Me:
"You're More *You* When You Drink!"

The Truth I Figured Out:
I'm More Me Than Ever Before

Have you ever recalled an embarrassingly drunk conversation you had with someone you barely knew and thought, "Well, at least I was being my most genuine self?" In those situations, you spoke and acted impulsively because alcohol hijacked your brain's ability to filter your reactions. Alcohol marketing boasts drinking as a solution to social anxiety, making us feel like we are more ourselves, or an even better version, when we're a few drinks deep. We've been led to believe that being drunk helps us get in tune with a more authentic side of ourselves. But all drinking does is numb your brain. There is nothing authentic about deadening the feelings in your body and mind.

Too often, though, we're told that drinking allows us to be more in the moment, to be more present, to be more authentic. My desperate need to be more authentic was most evident on the night I turned twenty-one, when I celebrated this milestone with my brother, Darron, in West Hollywood. Darron dared me to get a tattoo. I said no at least a dozen times, but six beers deep, I was no longer shy about taking on any challenge, let alone one from my brother. I agreed, and he and I stumbled into a local tattoo parlor, which was all too ready to tat me up, despite my obvious inebriation.

What was the tattoo, you ask? Just your typical thunder-throwing Zeus, or as I liked to call him, Colonial Sky Daddy. As if that weren't cringe-worthy enough, I got the tattoo on my right hip, directly above my butt. Hear me out. I was study-ing Greek mythology at the time, and my consciousness was

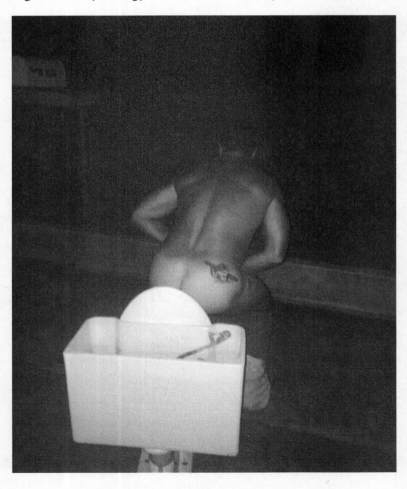

Finding humor in the journey! I'm baring it all, including my most vulnerable side.

definitely that of a separate, vengeful god. Because of some of my midwestern upbringing, I get a little nervous sometimes, thinking I am listening to the vindictive Colonial Sky Daddy version of god, and he will smite me by throwing a lightning bolt on my head, just as my tattoo depicts. Zeus, Colonial Sky Daddy, or whatever that fearmongering, judgmental, false, separate god is called these days, I curse you back! I cannot stand my tattoo. But it has served as a reminder to tell everyone, "Do *not* go out with a drunk Darron on your twenty-first birthday."

When I tell the story, everyone asks to see the tattoo. I am going to get it over with once and for all right here, so I can stop pulling my pants down in public. My goal with this book, and life in general, is to be as honest and vulnerable as possible. If this doesn't express my willingness to be vulnerable, I don't know what will. This photo was taken in Hawaii on a couple's night out, back when I was drinking. There was a toilet out on a curb to be picked up with the trash, and I pretended to use it.

Please do not reach for a drink to get the pain out of your eyes! I have to be the first ever to moon the reader in a self-help book. But, hey, whatever it takes to help wake you up from the Alcohol Matrix. Even shock therapy! My girls are already starting to tell their friends how embarrassing Daddy is, and I have told them it's my goal in their teenage years to embarrass them as much as possible. Girls, I honestly hope your friends never see this photo, *butt* if they do . . . hehehe! My girls are going to learn the truth about me, eventually, so I might as well reveal everything now— not only about me but also about their aunt and uncle, too, who similarly made a lot of mistakes trying to be their most authentic selves under the influence of alcohol.

About the only thing to do in our small midwestern town was to drink and cruise around the neighborhood. One night, my sister and her friends did just that. They drove to Sonic and purchased an extra-large drink of cola. Immediately, they dumped out half of the cup's contents on a patch of concrete by their car, then filled the half-empty cup with Seagram's Crown Royal, a midshelf Canadian whiskey that contains 35 percent alcohol. A few sips in, my sister needed to throw up. She stumbled toward the parking lot of a church so she could vomit in private. After puking her guts out, she wandered onto the shoulder of Route 66 in the middle of the night. She was alone, without a jacket, and very, very drunk.

After a few minutes, a large black truck pulled up. The driver asked if she needed a ride home. My sister's head was spinning, and her inhibitions, along with her sense of direction, were long gone. The man seemed friendly. She accepted his offer and hopped into his truck. You hear stories like this all the time, and they almost always end terribly. Fortunately, this one has a happy ending. He drove her home, then walked her up to our front door. He warned my sister to be more careful and tipped his hat to my mom, who was understandably furious at my sister. But she was also grateful and impressed with the young man. Turns out, my mother was right to be impressed. The young man was Garth Brooks, then a senior at our local high school.

Whether she realized it or not at the time, my sister had fallen for the myth that alcohol makes you more social. In her desire to fit in, she was inadvertently, but inevitably, pulled into the Alcohol Matrix. The next day, even sporting a brutal hangover, she had a great story to tell about getting picked up by a senior her first time drinking. Deep down, though, she knew she had also experienced the dark side of alcohol: left alone by her friends, she got sick and was nearly abducted on the side of the road. If Garth hadn't been such a nice guy, things could have ended very differently.

If your family drinks alcohol, they were probably the first ones to pull you into the Alcohol Matrix. But for most people, the teenage years are when the Alcohol Matrix is reinforced a hundredfold. I found this out at my friend's pool party. My sister found out in the parking lot of an Oklahoma Sonic. And my brother, Darron, found out in his childhood bedroom.

INTRODUCING ERNEST AND JULIO GALLO

Like me, Darron was never going to drink. He had experienced the trauma that alcohol causes up close and personal, and he swore he would never touch the stuff. He wasn't willing to risk it. But what he *was* willing to risk was hosting parties so his friends could get wasted. Because our mom was often gone on weekends and our two older sisters were away at college, Darron pretty much had the house to himself. I was usually at a friend's house. Darron, as a sophomore in high school, had the same small group of classmates since kindergarten, and our house became the group's clubhouse. At one party, a guy was hanging out, singing and playing guitar. Normally, the kid had a severe stutter, but when he sang, it didn't affect him. With his long perfect hair, striking blue eyes, and beautiful singing voice, the dude had girls lined up outside the door. Next to him was one of those big, puce-green glass jugs of Ernest and Julio Gallo white wine, which cost about five dollars and, according to Darron, sizzled in your mouth like a handful of Pop Rocks. As Darron tells it, he didn't know how he ended up in his room with this high school heartthrob, but Darron specifically remembers him asking if he could try some of his Ernest and Julio Gallo. Darron picked up the jug and started chugging. After four huge gulps, the teenage troubadour blurted out, without the hint of a stutter, "You're gonna make yourself throw up!"

When Darron finally lowered the bottle, he said with the

confidence of someone who had just found the key to life, "Ohhhh, I'm not gonna throw up."

And he didn't.

"What did happen," he told me later, "was that for the first time in my sixteen years on the planet, I felt 'right.' This was how life was supposed to be!"

He told me he felt a deep sense of relief. "Sparkles soon filled my vision, and the constant stream of horrible things I was always calling myself were suddenly quiet."

To this day, Darron swears he was addicted after that first drink. Maybe not to the alcohol, at least not yet. But that initial rush he felt standing in his bedroom definitely had him hooked. "It was like I had lived my entire life in a funhouse, where everything looked normal, but the floors slanted just enough that I would constantly stumble or slip. Then suddenly the floors corrected themselves, and I could walk with ease. It wasn't a struggle just to make it to the door."

His introduction to alcohol confirmed his unconscious programming, which reinforced the idea that alcohol is the perfect elixir, our most accessible painkiller. This allowed him to ignore the simmering symptoms of his child traumas and, as far as he was concerned, finally start being his most authentic self—the version of himself who felt "right" under the influence of alcohol. Like all of us, Darron grew up brainwashed by the cultural glamorization of alcohol, but his personal experience with it put the final nail in his concoction coffin. He swallowed it whole, then went deep into the Alcohol Matrix. Alcohol quickly became his way of life, just as it did with me.

Now, Darron and I are very different people. Very different. The funniest person I know, Darron went on to host a famous drag queen show in San Francisco's Castro neighborhood, which culminated in a national TV show. Despite our differences, he and I both became addicted to alcohol. It took me decades of moderate drinking to become addicted, but my brother became dependent almost immediately.

I'll get back to that in a second. For now, I want to talk about how peer pressure feeds into the Alcohol Matrix–inspired narrative that drinking, usually to excess, is not only expected but is the only way you can be true to yourself. In my experience, this way of thinking usually leads to some truly terrible decisions and, as I'm about to detail, some questionable, if not reckless, behavior, especially in young men.

I started drinking to fit in, or so I thought for the longest time. Everyone I knew in high school—jocks, nerds, my own siblings, and everyone in between—wanted to steal a few glugs from the bottle in their parents' bar cart or liquor cabinet. Classmates with older siblings who could buy booze were gods among mere mortals, and if you knew a liquor store that didn't check IDs, your info was as coveted as stock tips from a Wall Street insider. Everybody wanted to be invited to the party. Even if they had no interest in drinking prior to high school, it didn't take long to learn that alcohol was the key to getting in. Peer pressure is the primary reason most teenagers drink for the first time. If they don't drink, the thinking goes, they're nobody—a loser. And, as we all know, no one wants to be perceived as a nobody, especially a teenager who is still trying to figure out who they are.

Social media only exacerbates the pressure to fit in, which is just one of the reasons teenage drinking is becoming more common. Research—and, hell, even local news reports—tells us that highly emotional teens trying to discover their identities experience FOMO (fear of missing out) when they see their classmates on social media living it up with flasks at a music concert or standing around beer kegs at a house party. If they don't join the party right now, teens feel anxious, rejected, and unwanted. These social media posts create a bias that drinking is normal, misrepresenting what being a teenager is all about. From what I've seen, there aren't many examples of study sessions and college applications floating around TikTok. Meanwhile, the booze-ridden posts on Finstas (fake Instagram accounts, hidden from parents) positively affirm that alcohol and high school social success are synonymous. By the time teenagers enter college, many believe alcohol is the only way to make a lot of friends and the only chance to hook up. This is exactly what Darron and I believed, too, back in the pre-TikTok analog days of yore.

As I wrote in the first chapter, I used alcohol to summon the courage to talk to my high school sweetheart for the first time. By college, sex and alcohol went together like bread and butter. As I got older, sex and alcohol continued to comingle, and I reinforced the association between them. If I wanted sex, alcohol was almost always involved. Since I now have two gorgeous young daughters, I am going to hit this one hard with a few staggering stats:

- Among college undergraduate students, "26.4% of females and 6.8% of males experience rape or sexual assault through physical force, violence, or incapacitation."[1]

- A majority of sexual assaults involve alcohol or other substances.[2]

- Guys in college know that alcohol loosens inhibitions, and now, more girls in college are drinking on a monthly basis than guys.[3] The combination is a recipe for disaster, and the problem is only getting worse.

There is a scene in the classic movie *Animal House* in which two drunk college kids are making out. The girl is topless, and she passes out on the guy's bed. While he tries to figure out what to do, a devil and an angel appear on his right and left shoulders, offering advice. Should he take advantage of her, or should he take care of her? In the movie, the angel wins.

After a typical frat party, the conversation between guys probably sounds something like this:

"Did you and that one chick hook up?"

"Yeah, she was cool, but I can't remember her name."

And the first-year sorority girl says, "I think I hooked up with him. Or did I? I don't know."

Her rush captain replies, "Really? Whoops. I have been there. Do you like him? What are you going to do?"

"Not really. I'll just ghost him."

Guys hype each other up about who their targets are, and girls travel in squads so they can keep an eye on each other. Everyone gets drunk before the party so they can arrive "relaxed," which, if we're being honest, means uninhibited. We're programmed to think that parties are the best way to hook up. Alcohol greases the gears to make it happen. Guys often don't want to talk about this because it's uncomfortable to face how powerfully predatory their subconscious can be under the influence of hormones and alcohol. After I had my alcohol awakening, I realized how unconsciously, even unconscionably, I was behaving. I was completely controlled by a world of hormones and alcohol as a young man.

THE BUSINESS OF DRINKING

Sex isn't the only powerful force that keeps us plugged into the Alcohol Matrix, however. Success is almost as potent, and it stuck with me long after I left campus. Literally all of my bosses and sales managers have been big drinkers. Sharing a drink was the easiest way to get on their good side. If we could get drunk together, we could do business together. At least, that's how the myth went. And, in my experience, peer pressure at work is incredibly powerful because if you don't follow along with the crowd, you might lose out on a promotion, the big client, or your dream job. Corporate America doesn't just embrace drinking for men and women: it pushes it. It's a way to network with others in your field and prove that you "belong." People like to work with people similar to themselves. Having a difference in opinion over something as deeply ingrained as alcohol could turn you into an outsider. If you want to climb the ladder, the first rung starts at the bar. If you want to bond with your coworkers, why not bring a bottle to the office? If you want to sweeten the deal with your clients, take them out for drinks. Your company's treat, of course. In Japan, this kind of corporate behavior even has a name. The Japanese call a meeting with drinks "nomunication," a blend of the Japanese verb *nomu*, meaning "to drink," and the English word *communication*. It represents the breaking down of formal walls to connect with the person behind the title and the suit. In Japanese business culture, group harmony is incredibly important, so getting drunk during a business deal or after a meeting is commonplace.

After my first chug of beer in high school, I used and abused alcohol for years because every social environment I knew seemed to value alcohol and reward those who got drunk. I wanted to join the high school fun, so I drank. I wanted to hook up in college, so I drank. I wanted to celebrate the holidays, so I drank. I wanted to advance my career, so I drank. In every area of my life, I felt the need not only to fit in but also to stand out—to be seen as the quintessential life of the party. To be perfectly honest, I didn't know who I was without alcohol. Without it, I was lost and, if I didn't feel as if I were the life of the party, I simply didn't know what to do or how to act. Now, this didn't always mean I was dancing on a table with a lampshade on my head, but I definitely used alcohol as a way to get noticed. What ultimately hooked Darron into making alcohol his way of life was the way alcohol made him feel. What ultimately hooked me was how alcohol made me act.

There was a period of time, though, when I was alcohol-free. I was modeling, so I needed to look great and feel completely

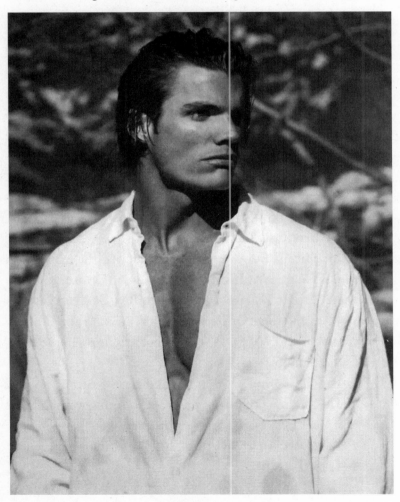

Fond memories of an adventurous photoshoot in an icy river outside of Milan. #Throwback

comfortable in my body. I laid off the beer and booze and meditated every day, but only because I needed to be in great shape. I wasn't anywhere near reckoning with my relationship with alcohol. All I knew was that I looked fantastic and felt incredible.

The only thing that mattered to me at that time in my life was that I was getting paid good money to model underwear. You couldn't drink alcohol and look good enough to get modeling jobs, so that is why I didn't drink.

It's amazing how fast I slipped right back into the alcohol-fueled lifestyle after my year of being alcohol-free, however. I had booked a gig in Milan, and an hour after I landed, jet-lagged and exhausted, I got a call from my agent asking me to go to a fashion show that evening. The iconic fashion designer Gianni Versace had recently been murdered at his South Beach mansion in Miami, and his sister, Donatella, was holding a colossal memorial show in his honor. I couldn't believe it—just moments after landing in Italy for the first time, I was already getting the opportunity to go to a show for one of fashion's most famous names.

When I arrived, I immediately felt insecure, self-conscious, and out of place: a horrible social cocktail. All the big fashion designers—Giorgio Armani, Miuccia Prada, Donna Karan—were there. I spotted Demi Moore, then Boy George, who was wearing a tiger-print top hat and thick mascara. Impeccably dressed models and VIPs were everywhere, done up in the latest high fashion, impossibly chic.

"Buona sera," purred a warm female voice. I turned to find myself face-to-face with one of the most stunning women I had ever seen. She had laser-sharp features but soft, big eyes. Her long, dark hair was rich and thick. She looked at me expectantly with an eyebrow raised.

"Uhm...hi." I replied awkwardly. "Sorry, I don't speak Italian."

A coy smile played across her lips. "Va bene," she said. "I speak some English. You like drink? You seem un po' nervoso."

I glanced around quickly. Everyone had a drink in their hand except for me. So, I nodded, "Si." The woman slid up to the nearby bar and returned with a martini in each hand. Suddenly, I was holding one, and our glasses were clinking together. The Alcohol Matrix assured me that since I had an alcoholic drink in my hand, I was as cool as everyone else.

I had been shoved back into the Alcohol Matrix far too easily.

Still, I thought I was on the path to making it big, and if alcohol was part of the deal, so be it. Some of the other models and I opted for vodka sodas, pretending we were cheating the system by getting drunk without the extra calories, even though there were one hundred extra calories in every shot. I didn't want to be the person other people were afraid to invite out or acted awkward around because I wouldn't drink. I wanted to be fun, cool, social, and fearless.

SOCIAL OR ANTISOCIAL?

Whether you fell into the Alcohol Matrix in high school or in college or somehow managed to avoid it until you entered the workforce, you have most likely found yourself in so-called social situations in which you weren't exactly at your best. That's what the examples above demonstrate, regardless of when or where they took place. Alcohol loves to tell us that it empowers us to be the life of the party, or at least an enthusiastic participant. The irony is that in the very situations we're supposed to be most social, we too often end up exhibiting antisocial and self-destructive behavior.

As you probably guessed by now, I know this all too well. But don't just take my word for it. A recent study found that excessive alcohol consumption increases _antisocial_ behavior, or a dysfunctional way of perceiving situations and other people, which causes you to act in an aggressive or intimidating manner. Under normal (i.e., alcohol-free) conditions, people usually stop demonstrating antisocial behavior with age, usually around the end of puberty. What this study found, though, is the opposite. Alcohol consumption by young people (under fifteen years old) leads to them engaging in higher than usual antisocial behavior.[4] What's more is that according to another study, the prevalence of antisocial personality disorder and syndromal adult antisocial behavior was, respectively, 4.3 percent and 20.3 percent. This was highest among men, especially white or Native American young men who are unmarried, less educated, and earning less than the average American. Both antisocial syndromes, the study noted, were "significantly associated with 12-month and lifetime substance use" as well as other psychological and emotional disorders, including "dysthymia/persistent depressive, bipolar I, posttraumatic stress and borderline and schizotypal personality disorders."[5]

Although I do like to make light of my own experiences, this is hardly a laughing matter. Nearly a quarter of men today exhibit some kind of antisocial behavior, and our cultural reverence for alcohol consumption is accelerating this devastating trend.

Here's a more encouraging study, which not only blew my mind but also let me know I was onto something as I made the necessary switch from alcohol to easy-to-find nonalcoholic beverages and mocktails. A meta-analysis in the journal *Psychology of Addictive Behaviors* showed that people are more social when they are given a placebo than when they are given actual alcohol.[6] That's right: when test subjects were given placebo cocktails at a bar, 99 percent of them reported that they consumed real alcohol, felt the effects of intoxication, and had an amazing time socializing. Jokes were flying, smiles beamed, and inhibitions were lowered, yet there was no addictive, toxic poison flowing through their veins. Placebo participants did not slobber on their neighbors, make insensitive comments, or lose focus midconversation like the drinking group did. Mocktails provided all the social benefits of "drinking" with none of the drawbacks, and the study found that people who didn't consume alcohol found the night *more* enjoyable. I wish I'd known about this study when I was in Milan, or South Beach, or Liverpool, or Oklahoma, or anywhere, really.

This study shows that you can still fit in without alcohol. You can still stand out. You can still get that promotion you're after. And, yes, you can still be the life of the party. Most importantly, this study shows that you don't need alcohol to be your most authentic self. In fact, as I hope you understand by now, alcohol is more likely keeping you from finding and expressing your most authentic self.

CHAPTER 3

The Lie Alcohol Told Me:
"You're Doing Great!"

The Truth I Figured Out:
I Was at My Worst

After earning my master's degree in psychology, I worked in the ten-dollar-an-hour mental health field, the first step in finishing my doctorate and going through the very long process of earning my license to practice. Instead of putting in my requisite hours, though, I quit and took a sales job in corporate America, which basically required little more from me than getting drunk and playing golf with the CEO on gorgeous courses all around the world. I was having a blast, and I was loath to give up the fun.

But, out of the blue, I got a call from Ryan Seacrest's crew in 2009. They were in search of a telegenic male with a doctorate in psychology for a new reality television show called *LA Shrink*. The role was simple: talk to aspiring and wannabe celebrities. About their problems. On cable television.

Hollywood picked me out of the crowded field of mental health professionals because of three letters—PhD. Even I had to admit, though, that those three letters were a touch misleading. Although I had put in the blood, sweat, and tears to earn every bit of my master's degree, by the time I began writing my doctoral dissertation, I was drinking and really didn't care any-more. I ended up copying and pasting part of my master's thesis into my dissertation. You'll notice that I didn't put those three letters after my name on the cover of this book. I choose not to use those letters with my name at all, not just because I didn't put in the full effort on my dissertation, but also because those letters immediately imply that the person who has them knows more than the person who doesn't. All these years later, I still don't use those three little letters. Instead, I prefer to paraphrase Socrates: all I know is I know nothing.

Around the time the Seacrest crew reached out to me, how-ever, I was so laser focused on drinking every night that I hardly cared about anything else. Because I was still entirely consumed by my own ego, however, I made sure to include those three important letters after my name, on anything I could—my résumé, my email signature, my *Men's Health* magazine sub-scription, and my social media accounts. Stalking my digital presence, the Seacrest team found what they were looking for: a male model with a PhD.

Let's just say I was interested. *Very* interested.

In the mid-aughts, Ryan Seacrest was quickly becoming one of the most powerful producers in Hollywood. The host of *Ameri-can Idol*, a cultural phenomenon, he was a household name. His star, which was already shining brighter than the midday sun, was still very much on the rise. Industry leaders were calling him the next Dick Clark, and everyone wanted to team up with him in his early forays into producing, me included. But I wanted to be honest, which meant I had to tell his team that I didn't have a license to practice. They didn't care. And, after less than a week in Hollywood, during which time I taped a few interviews on camera, I was called to meet with the man himself.

Things were moving fast, but as I quickly learned, no matter how long I had to prepare, nothing could have gotten me ready for the harsh truth about reality television. My first hint that there are two kinds of reality occurred even before I had a chance to sit down with Ryan Seacrest. While I was sitting in the waiting room at Ryan Seacrest Productions, a ripped, short, very good-looking guy walked in. He was wearing a black felt hat, black leather vest, and—yup—black leather pants. Silver chains dangled off him from head to toe. The four women in the room came to serious attention. When the guy winked at the receptionist, she blushed and grinned like a schoolgirl.

Who is this guy? I thought.

He flopped down in the chair next to me.

"Hey," he said.

"Hey," I said back.

He looked me up and down, and I could tell he was trying to figure out who I was and whether I was important. That's when it hit me. This was Dave Navarro: guitarist, singer, songwriter, actor, and TV personality.

"What's your name?" he asked.

"Dustin . . . and you're Dave, right?"

"Yup, are you waiting to see Ryan?"

I nodded.

"Well," he said, "you are going to have to wait until I'm done."

There is a serious hierarchy in Hollywood. I learned very quickly that I was not at Mr. Navarro's level, and even though my appointment with Ryan was scheduled before his (if he even had one), I was to wait my turn—rock gods and pop stars came before us plebes and regular folks.

After thirty minutes of listening to the women in the room talk about how "short but still so freaking hot" Dave was, I was finally allowed to go to Ryan's office.

Ryan greeted me with a big hug. He is a welcoming, friendly

guy and immediately put me at ease. "So, you're Dustin. Everyone tells me we look a lot alike, and now that I see you in person,
I think so, too."

I smiled and deadpanned, "I know, I get people asking me if I
am you all the time. Do you get me?"

"Uh . . . no," he said, thinking I was serious.

I wasn't at Seacrest's level either.

A woman came into the office, and Ryan told her, "This is
Dustin. He is our new LA Shrink." Then he asked me, "How old
are you, Dustin?"

I was shaken by the news that I had gotten the job, but managed to reply, "Thirty-seven."

Ryan nodded his head and said to the woman, "I'm four years
younger, so this is what I will look like in four years."

The woman, who I later found out was the coproducer, laughed
and shook her head. "You wish!" she said.

She gave my damaged Hollywood ego the exact boost it
needed.

I could tell that she was on the same level as Ryan. He was a
little hurt by her messing with him. But his bruised ego didn't
stop him. He continued the meeting without missing a beat,
merrily as ever and a complete professional, which is probably
one of the many reasons he's so successful. That, and another
crucial element: he's present, always in the moment. I can't speak
more highly of a person than Ryan Seacrest. He reminds me a bit
of my ex-wife. They both have a natural ability to listen to others
with genuine compassion and empathy. That's truly a gift. Few
people have it. The best spouses, friends, counselors, interview-
ers, and radio/TV hosts don't just ask great questions; they are
great listeners. Think about how easily Ryan talks with celebrities. Or other great interviews, like Terry Gross or even Howard
Stern. Though all three evince wildly different personality types,

they are all great listeners, which is why they're able to get their guests to open up so freely. They are all so present.

For the pilot, producers taped me interviewing girlfriends of celebrities, fame-chasing hangers-on, and daughters of Hollywood A-listers. I tried to teach them how they could improve their troubled lives in the limelight. Unfortunately, I was a complete hypocrite. On set, I was talking to Kanye West's then-girlfriend, evaluating her mental, physical, and emotional health in between her trips with Kanye to visit the Cannes Film Festival or Coachella. Then, once we wrapped for the week, I was flying to Vegas, where I did nothing but get hammered and party in penthouse hotel rooms. On Monday morning, I was always back for my 9 a.m. call, ready to play the role of the healthy doctor.

The women I analyzed in front of the camera were as uninterested in a healthier lifestyle as I was. They were in Hollywood for the nonstop party of endless martinis and ecstasy pills. Trust me, a twentysomething claiming she'll clean up her life in ten years has no desire to pump the brakes on Kanye's lifestyle. She's not suddenly going to tell him that although she very much wants to go the Grammys with him, or an exclusive Hollywood party at Jamie Foxx's house, she wants to attend them alcohol-free. Because the producers similarly knew that wouldn't sell, they had no interest in me telling these young women, "Maybe ease off on the drinks and tell Kanye you need a personal day." They wanted me to keep the drama at a manic level and keep the dream of the nonstop party alive, knowing that fans everywhere would eat up the insane celebrity culture that conditions us to live like there's no tomorrow. Despite my hypocrisy, I still didn't like the message I was sending; but that was fine, because *LA Shrink* was soon cancelled.

But I wasn't finished in reality television. They still wanted me to "help" people. This time in Dallas. After acting as the *LA*

Shrink, I transformed into the *Dallas Life Coach*. The producers at Endemol shipped me and the film crew from Hollywood to Dallas, where instead of starlets and models I "counseled" trust-fund babies and the daughters of billionaire oil tycoons, trying to get them to "turn their lives around." My job was to conduct "therapy sessions" with these women, but it was the same story as *LA Shrink*. After shooting a scene in a club, we'd buy the whole crowd a round of drinks, and people would fling themselves at me, offering drinks, drugs, sex, and an invite to the after-party. I partied with Mark Cuban at the Dallas Mavericks facilities, woke up half-drunk at some other billionaire's mansion, and acted like a put-together doctor on reality TV later that day. They seriously dressed me up in cowboy boots and a ridiculous hat, threw me on a horse, and fed me lines right before shouting "Action!" It was total chaos, a complete deception—exactly what the producers wanted. It didn't matter that the scenes were completely scripted. It was a purposely produced deception, and audiences generally ate it up, whether they were in on the con or not. It was entertainment, pure and simple, a vehicle for selling products and a specific lifestyle. The more outlandish and destructive, the better.

Like *LA Shrink*, though, *Dallas Life Coach* was cancelled. Ultimately, MTV decided to run a different show in our time slot, another reality show about some bridge-and-tunnel kids who loved to party at the beach—without a meddlesome therapist getting in their way. It was called *Jersey Shore*.

I don't blame celebrities at all for struggling with any kind of addiction. It's incredibly difficult to live a healthy lifestyle when everyone around you is in the middle of a nonstop, world-class party, and drinks, drugs, and sex are everywhere, all the time. The people on TV who tell us to live free, party hard, and stay young forever are merely reading their lines. And these lines are always the same—that no matter what they get up to, that no matter how bad things might get, they're always doing great. They say these lines because they want you to feel the same thing. No matter how bad things may be because of your drinking, you're doing great. If they ever stopped saying these scripted lines, they'd have to consider how they really feel. And I'm sure they'd admit that they weren't doing so great.

THE SHOW MUST GO ON

Here's a quick story about Darron and his misadventures with fame. Darron will be the first to tell you that he never wanted to be a drag queen, per se. Of course, he'll also tell you that he never wanted to get addicted to alcohol, but things happen. Sometimes you end up with an addiction to alcohol, like me. Other times, you end up so desperate for attention and applause that you find yourself onstage dressed in women's clothing, like Darron. And sometimes you get both.

My brother always loved Lily Tomlin, Carol Burnett, and Jonathan Winters and the amazing show *Greater Tuna,* with all the characters they created and played. After moving to San Francisco, he wanted to do something like that, so in the years before YouTube, he started a public access show about this country woman who hosts a white-trash cooking show out of her mobile home. He got a producer, built a set, and wrote a bunch of scripts. He was ready to go, except he didn't have any other actors to play the different parts, including the show's hostess, a character he called Wenda Watch. In true Darron fashion, he said, "Screw it. I'll play all the characters!" He slapped on a wig, some white cat-eye glasses (an homage to Vera Carp of *Greater Tuna*), made some lipstick do triple duty as lipstick, rouge, and eyeshadow, and put on a dress that he had to duct tape together in the back because he couldn't zip it up.

His show was a hit, and Darron was getting invitations to perform at various events. Eventually, he hosted a weekly show at a bar in the Castro called Harvey's, named after Harvey Milk. The show ran for two years, all while Darron was drinking heavily.

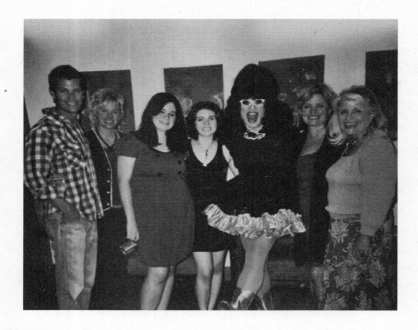

Celebrating love and individuality with my amazing family.

"I was able to keep it together at first," he told me. "I wouldn't have a drink until I was at the bar. Then I started having one or two while getting ready. I didn't have to drive since I only lived three blocks from Harvey's, or as I used to call it, 'staggering distance.' What I thought was the greatest thing ever, but now know was a curse, was that I got free drinks at the bar."

Darron also got free drinks at other clubs where he performed.

"People always loved to buy me drinks as well, because nothing shushes that gnawing knowledge in the back of your mind that keeps saying, 'You're drinking too much, you have a problem' like a big ol' sloppy, sloshed drag queen. One look at me, and everyone else was like, 'Oh, I'm doing great!'"

Away from the spotlight, Darron was struggling, usually just to get home. After one particularly hard-drinking night, he left the club in the middle of the show to run back to his house to get a Dolly Parton CD because someone requested one of her songs. He was so drunk that he walked out of his own show. The next morning, he didn't really "wake up" so much as he "came to." He had managed to get his girdle and three layers of tights down, but not quite off. He still wore one silver cowboy boot, his wig was askew, like a side ponytail, and a fake eyelash was stuck to his cheek.

"If this wasn't the bottom," he told me, "I don't know what was. I couldn't get any lower. Or so I thought. I reached down into my purse—one of those deep, wide numbers with a jeweled peacock on the side—to get a cigarette but instead pulled out . . . wait for it . . . an entire roast chicken."

He had an entire rotisserie chicken from one of those grocery store chrome heat lamp cases in his purse. Eventually, he pieced together what happened. He remembered losing his tips on the way home. He also remembered needing to urinate, and rather than finishing his three-block walk to his apartment, he decided to sneak behind a giant dumpster of a Cala Foods grocery store. Apparently, after relieving himself, he had a hankering for some supermarket chicken. Without any money, he went into Cala Foods, covered in his own piss, and decided to steal an entire rotisserie chicken. Not a candy bar or can of soup. Not an apple or even a deli sandwich. But an entire hot chicken. And this was his local store. He shopped there all the time! "So, this either means that I somehow took the chicken from the warmer and got it into my purse and got out of there with no one noticing the extra-large, kleptomaniacal, and apparently incontinent man in a dress with a chicken in his purse, or, and I'm assuming this is more likely the case, they did see me steal the chicken and were like, 'I'm not messin' with her.'"

I asked Darron if he considered quitting drinking after this.

"No, honey. I peeled the eyelash from my cheek and the wig from my head. Then, with tights still around my ankles, I hop, hop, side-shuffled to the kitchen, poured me a big glass of warm, boxed white Zinfandel, and made purse-chicken sandwiches for me and my roommates."

Like the reality stars I was "helping," Darron believed he was doing great because that's what we're supposed to believe. Heck, I still believed the same thing, even though I was partying all night before I showed up on set as a professional therapist trying to help aspiring starlets get their collective shit together. And they showed up on set with me, after partying all night, to say how committed they were to making changes. Darron, me, the reality stars—we were all doing great. That's what we told ourselves and each other, because if we didn't, like any scripted show, the entire story would fall apart if we started asking too many questions about the pretty obvious holes in the plot.

Darron and I continued drinking for years, and life carried on. From the outside looking in, I seemed to be thriving. My now ex-wife and I met at a sushi bar one night. We didn't exchange numbers, but about six months later, we ran into each other at a wine bar and became inseparable for twelve years. In 2008, the Great Recession hit, and she and I packed up and started working remotely, living around the world. We were digital nomads. I sold health insurance, and she was an account executive for a mortgage company. We were both super successful. We invested our money in real estate, which enabled me to retire in 2022.

And yet for all of my seeming good fortune, I wasn't ready to confront reality. Neither was Darron. You already know where my drinking took me: in the back of a police car, hands zip-tied behind my back, and my face smushed against the plexiglass partition. In addition to shoplifting a rotisserie chicken, Darron was charged with two DUIs. He got off on the first because the cops didn't read him his rights. But his second DUI put him in an Oklahoma jail cell over Thanksgiving weekend. Darron was also celebrating his birthday, which happened to land on Thanksgiving that year. He was on a bender, drinking day and night. When he ran out of liquor, he drove to the liquor store and bought a bottle of Old Crow, a cheap rotgut. Bending down to pick it up, he fell over. The owner helped him up, then sold him the whiskey, before helping him into his car. Then she called the cops. They arrested Darron in his driveway. By the time he got booked, all the judges had already gone for the holiday weekend. He spent close to a week in jail, tossed into a cell with an alleged pedophile and attempted murderer because Oklahoma still classified gay men as sexual deviants.

Before I ever got involved with reality television, I worked at a crisis intervention clinic. One of my first intakes was a man who was addicted to alcohol. For years, he was abusing alcohol in an attempt to alleviate his depression. Like me, he couldn't confront reality and used alcohol as an escape. When he showed up, it was my first week, and I went through the motions of checking him in, doing all the paperwork, and getting to know him and his medical history. After talking with him for a while, I led him up to his room, but I did not thoroughly search through all of his personal belongings like I was supposed to. I regret to say that I forgot to check his toiletry bag, even though he told me he was suicidal.

Later that night, he went to the bathroom with the razor that I should have taken away from him. He might not have lived through the night if we hadn't seen the blood seeping into the hallway under the door. I went cold at the sight of the pooling blood. My heart started racing as I busted through the door with a colleague. Blood was everywhere. I saw everything at once. The razor, the wound, his body unconscious and slumped against the wall. It's an image I'll never forget. I didn't pause for a moment until the ambulance took him away. Everything up to that point was pure shock and action as we rushed to stop the bleeding, call the hospital, and keep the rest of the facility under control.

Does this man's story read like he was doing great? Or what about Darron's story? Or what about my own? I don't know about you, but when I read these specific accounts—and many others like them—I see only heartrending horrors of men trapped in their addiction, at the worst points of their lives.

TIMELINE: TWO WEEKS ALCOHOL-FREE

After two weeks of being alcohol-free, the majority of people will begin to feel really good and more alive as brain fog and lethargy wear off. Your body will thank you every day for not poisoning yourself with alcohol by returning to its natural state of better digestion, workout recovery, hydration, and energy. Your mood and sleep quality will consistently improve. You'll feel excited to get going in the morning instead of feeling groggy. You'll no longer struggle to drag yourself out of bed when your alarm goes off. More subtle improvements can surface as well, ranging from sharper eyesight to increased attention.

On average, alcohol detox takes between seven and ten days, so most of the alcohol and its nasty byproducts have left your body after a week. But even when the alcohol toxins are gone, the physical and psychological healing process will take a few more months. Stick to the healthy habits you began over the last two weeks. Now that the alcohol-free benefits are abundant, you'll really be able to feel the difference a healthy diet and regular exercise are making for your mind and body.

During my second week without alcohol, I started craving sweets and chocolate, which makes sense because my body was used to all those sugary calories (remember, your body converts alcohol into sugar). Don't feel guilty for indulging in dessert at the end of a meal instead of having alcohol. I eat a lot more desserts now and still keep the weight off because I'm not consuming empty alcohol calories. Just be sure you're not using food in a compulsive way to comfort any underlying mental health issues that may surface once you stop drinking.

At the same time, your body is starting to heal. Your digestive system is improving because alcohol-induced inflammation decreases and healthy gut bacteria starts to flourish. Because years of consistent drinking leaves your body damaged, however, some organs take longer to repair than others. One such organ is the brain. Consistently soaking your brain in alcohol causes it to shrink and lose functionality. But after two weeks of being alcohol-free, the brain starts its regrowth process, filling in the gaps left by alcohol consumption and vitamin deficiencies. These repairs lead to better motor skills, improved memory, and overall sharper cognitive ability.

After about two weeks of being alcohol-free, there is a high occurrence of relapse, so be on close guard for any cravings or "Alcohol benefits me" thoughts that may come up. Two weeks in, you haven't created a new habit yet, and your old compulsive drinking habit is still in force. Plan ahead for what you will do when your mind tries to follow the familiar path of grabbing a drink so you can quickly reroute to a healthy new habit like exercise, meditation, or even just calling a friend.

Psychological issues become more pronounced at this time as well, which could be a withdrawal symptom or the emergence of a preexisting problem that no longer has alcohol suppressing it. If you have any mental anxiety, depression, or pain arise, get professional help.

PART II

ALCOHOL, CULTURE, AND THE COLLECTIVE UNCONSCIOUS

CHAPTER 4

The Lie Alcohol Told Me:
"You Know What You're Doing"

The Truth I Figured Out:
I Was Blind to the Truth

Throughout most of my life, I believed I was getting away with something, that I had somehow figured out how to outsmart the system. I had traveled the world, made a lot of money, and had some cool adventures with international models and Hollywood celebrities. Even if things didn't end up exactly the way I wanted—with endless fame and generational wealth, for starters—I still felt as if I had made out more than okay. Much more so than that goofy-looking teenager awkwardly handling a shotgun ever thought possible.

Looking back now, though, I can clearly see some of the warning signs I originally overlooked or willfully ignored, the same ones trying to alert me to the fact that things weren't as stable as I thought. Like the time Darron watched me pack up my car for yet another adventure with my family in a new city. I was getting a head start on our move. My then-wife and our daughters were going to fly to Myrtle Beach, South Carolina, to meet me after I had a chance to set things up for us. My car was already crammed tight with our stuff—boxes, suitcases, and other domestic sundries. But I still had to fit in two more things: a car seat and a case of wine. Only one would fit, I quickly realized, and I stood in my driveway trying to make what felt like the most consequential decision of the day.

"Just leave the wine," Darron told me, laughing about my dilemma.

"I don't know, man. It's pretty good wine. It's expensive, too."

I weighed my options for a moment.

"You know, I could always just buy another car seat when I get to Myrtle Beach."

Darron looked at me the same way the Grail Knight in *Indiana Jones and the Last Crusade* looked at the villain when he drank from the wrong cup before getting turned into dust. "He chose poorly."

Now, Darron had made more than his share of poor decisions, particularly about alcohol. So, I thought he was laughing along with me when he shouted, "Screw the car seat! He's taking the booze!"

I probably should have picked up on his sarcasm, which in retrospect was about as subtle as his drag show in the Castro.

"I totally understood why you picked the wine," Darron later told me, "because I'd made similar decisions myself. But that was actually the second red flag I spotted the morning of your little driveway dilemma."

"What was the first?" I asked.

"The first was the simple fact that you were traveling with a *case* of wine. Not a bottle or two! An entire case!"

Point taken, older brother. But that morning in the driveway, four years away from my final midflight Bloody Mary, I was still under the illusion that everything was going great. I still believed that I was fully aware of what I was doing, that all of the decisions I made, all of the emotions I felt, and all of the ways in which

I behaved were of my own volition. Even if they weren't always received in the way I had intended, I could always assure myself that they at least made sense to me, inside my thirty-plus-year-old brain.

At that point in my life, standing in the driveway, I might have thought I was outsmarting the system, but I can admit now that I didn't even know how the system worked. I wasn't the iconoclast I liked to imagine in my head, forging my own way while everyone else obeyed the rules and followed normal conventions. No, I was just another captive of the Alcohol Matrix, held there by the unconscious allure of alcohol, the same unconscious allure that exists virtually within all of us.

THE COLLECTIVE UNCONSCIOUS

This might seem like a digression, but I want to tell you about my love of aspen trees, my favorite kind of tree. I've always loved the white bark, which is starkly gorgeous in the afternoon sun and in the early-evening gloam. I've also always loved how an aspen's leaves turn gold in the fall, a colorful explosion above its white core. The most interesting thing about aspens, though, is how they are all connected at the roots. Although they look like separate trees, a group of them is considered one organism. In fact, the Pando aspen grove in Utah is the largest single organism in the world.[1] Now, what does this have to do with the Alcohol Matrix? This is exactly how the collective unconscious works: timeless roots, deep below our conscious awareness, connect every human who has ever lived or will ever live. Because we're all connected, we pass on physical traits, cultural instincts, and ways of thinking between generations. Some are specific to individual families and their descendants, but others are universal across humankind. Carl Jung referred to these widespread, learned thought patterns as the *collective unconscious*, humankind's own forest of aspen trees![2]

The collective unconscious—the inherited psychological foundation shared by all human beings—is considered to be one of Jung's most important ideas. He realized that members of society share certain ways of thinking that go unnoticed because they are taken for granted. These thought patterns take place beyond the level of conscious awareness. Most of the time we disregard them, but whether or not we pay attention to them, they continue to influence us every day. Facial expressions, for instance. They are common to all humans, regardless of ethnicity or era. Smiling is a universal expression of happiness, whereas scowling is a universal expression of aggression. No one taught you to understand this relationship; you just knew it. This web of ideas, customs, and stereotypes bombards you before you even speak a language. Psychologists refer to these fundamental belief structures as preverbal, and they are especially difficult to reprogram. For the most part, this isn't a problem, because the ideas passed down to us in the collective unconscious are often positive and helpful. If something smells bad and tastes off, don't eat it—or drink it.

This is evident in a study by Emory University where they wafted a cherry blossom smell to mice and at the same time gave them an electric shock. Generations of mice later reacted with anxiety and fear to the odor without ever encountering it before.[3]

However, certain ideas in the collective unconscious are harmful and can hold you back. Think about the narrative our culture subtly teaches us about gender roles. One recent analysis of popular children's clothing retailers found that boys' clothing almost exclusively contained depictions of *predatory* animals (lions, alligators, and dinosaurs), whereas girls' clothing was filled with *prey* animals (bunnies, butterflies, and ponies).[4] Another study on films found that female characters speak less than half as many lines as male characters, even in movies where the main character is female.[5] Thankfully, many people are starting to wake up to the biased messages that are fed to us through the collective unconscious. But we don't give the same attention to the messages we receive about alcohol. Stats suggest Americans are guzzling more beer, wine, and liquor than in our country's history.[6] And we're so amused by our favorite pastime, we trade funny memes about it or come up with kitschy slogans for our excessive drinking, like "I Don't Get Drunk, I Get Awesome." Or "Why Limit Happiness to One Hour?" Or "It's Wine O'Clock."

As clever as you might think these lines are, let me tell you, they're not exactly new. Silly memes and catchy slogans about alcohol have been around since at least 25,000 years before the birth of Christ! You think a drunk guy's stories are old? Let's take a quick look at how old our references to alcohol are.

Perhaps the earliest known representation of alcohol is the Venus of Laussel, an imaged carved on a cave wall in France that many scholars say dates back to the Paleolithic Era. The Paleolithic Venus appears to be holding a bison horn, which many scholars interpret as a reference to alcohol.[7] All the way on the other side of the world, in a village in northern China, archaeologists found a bunch of jars (or *kui*) that date back to 7,000 BC. Chemical analysis of the jars revealed that they held an alcoholic drink made of grapes, berries, and honey.[8] The oldest verified beer brewery was found in Israel, in a thirteen-thousand-year-old cave used for burials and death rites. Residue on stone containers found in the cave suggest the Israelites drank an alcoholic solution produced from wheat and barley for their rituals.[9] And I used to think my hometown had a rich history!

The *Code of Hammurabi*, one of the oldest known written works in existence, regularly mentions alcohol. One law describes the punishment for a tavern keeper who overcharges for drinks. When I was addicted to alcohol, I probably would have endorsed corporal punishment for such an egregious offense. Similarly, in the *Epic of Gilgamesh*, an ancient Sumerian tale written around the year 2,100 BC, a barmaid advises the hero to give up his search for the meaning of life and relax with a good beer instead. I'm pretty sure I dated a descendant of this barmaid in college. In Egypt, Cleopatra levied a beer tax to pay for her war with Rome. With beer sales doing well at the time, she didn't think this would be a problem. However, beer was also a popular medical remedy and was prescribed for more than a hundred different ailments. People didn't react well to their ruler taxing this "vital and important medicine."

The Greek poet Euripides was among the first to expose the risks of alcohol abuse. His play *Bacchae* portrayed followers of the god Bacchus committing a murder after drinking to excess. His work was not taken as a warning against the dangers of alcohol, however. Instead, the Roman Empire outlawed the play. Not alcohol, the play. By 200 BC in Rome, the production of wine was a standardized industry, and winemakers could distribute their product in bulk quantities.

In traditional Chinese medicine, alcohol was considered to have spiritual importance. Many of the important ceremonies in religious life involved alcohol in some way, including sacrifices, burial ceremonies, prayers, births, and oaths of allegiance. The eighth-century Chinese poet Li Bo, a known partaker of intoxicants, wrote extensively about the mystical qualities of alcohol. Persian mystics such as the Sufis and poet Omar Khayyam seem to have been influenced by Chinese philosophy via the Silk Road, heavily incorporating wine into their poetry, ideas, and religious beliefs between the twelfth and fourteenth centuries.

Although the Quran forbids even a drop of alcohol, the Torah and the Bible speak highly of drinking. In the Torah, alcohol is recommended to treat depression, illness, and pain. In the Bible, Jesus performs a miracle by changing water into wine.

Beyond its cultural significance, alcohol has played a central role in the political and legalistic development of the modern nation-state. This is when our unconscious understanding of alcohol as a central part of life was codified and set in place, like a keystone in a massive prison, the kind that keeps us captive to the cultural allure of alcohol today.

In medieval Europe, alcohol was an everyday drink. Knights and serfs, progenitors of my rugby mates outside of Liverpool, consumed low-strength alcohol in large amounts, probably because English ale was often safer than the country's supply of contaminated water. Drinking started to get out of hand. In the 1500s, English writers like Thomas Nash expressed a growing concern with alcohol addiction. Public perception of alcohol started to shift. For the first time in world history, public intoxication was outlawed. By 1606, the English Parliament passed an act to "Repress the Odious and Loathsome Sin of Drunkenness." Three decades later, in 1643, Parliament passed a new liquor tax, hoping to reduce the country's out-of-control alcohol consumption. The tax had the opposite effect. Increasing the price of alcohol led people to start brewing and distilling alcohol at home, which gave them even more (and cheaper) opportunities to drink. Other European countries developed their own home-brewed liquor to avoid taxation, which is how gin production began in Holland and whiskey got so popular in Ireland and Scotland.

When colonists fled Europe for America, they brought their taste for ale with them. Homebrewing was outlawed in New England in the middle of the seventeenth century. A labor strike reversed the law, and consumption continued to rise. George Washington famously considered alcohol a necessary prerequisite to the existence of an army. He was even in favor of erecting public distilleries to make alcohol a basic right, guaranteed to all Americans. When the newly formed American Congress levied a tax on whiskey in 1791, an organized resistance emerged, which forced Thomas Jefferson to repeal the unpopular tax ten years later when he was president.[10] As America grew into its own, so did a growing anti-alcohol effort among ministers and churches. The temperance movement started in the early 1800s and garnered a following called the Cold Water Army. These objectors didn't protest against alcohol in its entirety, just against drunkenness. In fact, most of them actually used alcohol during their services and consumed it regularly. Thus, drunkenness became a sin even while alcohol was an accepted part of everyday life, a viewpoint still very much alive today.

By 1860, the average American was estimated to drink nearly six gallons of pure alcohol per year, and the United States produced almost ninety million gallons of liquor annually. That's nearly three times as many gallons as the average American consumes today.[11]

By the early 1900s, concerns over America's increasing dependence on alcohol continued to grow. World War I prompted a temporary prohibition of alcohol, but Americans continued to drink after the Armistice. On December 18, 1917, the United States Senate proposed a constitutional amendment to prohibit alcohol. Less than two years later, in October 1919, Congress passed the Volstead Act (otherwise known as the National Prohibition Act), which articulated the rules for enforcing the ban on alcohol and defined the types of alcoholic beverages to be prohibited. The 18th Amendment was ratified on January 16, 1919. A year later, Prohibition officially started at midnight on January 17, 1920.[12] Americans resisted and continued to consume bootlegged alcohol in speakeasies across the country. In March 1933,

President Franklin Roosevelt signed the Cullen–Harrison Act, an amendment to the Volstead Act, which allowed manufacturers to start producing beer and wine. By the end of the year, Congress ratified the 21st Amendment, which repealed the 18th Amendment, and ended Prohibition.

EARLY RESEARCH AND EDUCATION

It wasn't until the late 1940s that the dangers of alcohol addiction were brought back to public attention. Physicians researched methods of curing alcohol dependence, and treatment centers opened throughout the country. With the aid of scientific research, alcohol education and addiction prevention became available to health-conscious Americans. In the 1970s, further research demonstrated that alcohol affects more than the drinkers. Prevalent studies linking car crash fatalities to drunk driving prompted the formation of alcohol-awakened associations such as Mothers Against Drunk Driving (MADD). In many states, legislators reduced the legal limit from 0.10 percent to 0.08 percent blood alcohol content while heightening penalties for drunk driving.

Still, we've only recently figured out what it means, physiologically, to be drunk. What actually happens to the body and brain while drinking alcohol? When alcohol is absorbed into the human body, it deadens and numbs the nervous system, including both your peripheral nerves (in your limbs) and your central nervous system (your brain and spinal cord). That's why it temporarily alleviates pain.

The conflicting ideas of alcohol as both healthy medicine and sinful vice have gone back and forth for millennia. This conflict between positive and negative ideations of the same concept is known as *cognitive dissonance*—a fancy way of saying your head isn't getting along with itself. This state of inconsistent thinking can lead to feelings of dissatisfaction, distress, and a desire to alter your behavior to reduce the internal conflict. However, the Alcohol Matrix inhibits our ability to resolve our dissonant thoughts and feelings. Instead, we drink alcohol to quiet these thoughts and feelings, rather than addressing them.

When I was trying to figure out how to get the case of wine and my daughter's car seat in the car, I was wrestling with this cognitive dissonance. Sure, it was a bit extreme, but I couldn't separate my unconscious and cultural understanding of alcohol with the very real conscious responsibilities of parenting and adulthood. The next time you're suffering from cognitive dissonance, when you can't wrap your head around your own head, I want you to think of me in my driveway, standing over a case of wine and my daughter's car seat, trying to figure out a solution, as if I were a judge considering a passage from the *Code of Hammurabi.*

Look, we're all caught between these two poles. Many of us have woken up with a disgusting hangover after a night on the town, praying to the porcelain god, swearing we'll never drink again. Yet, when Friday night comes around, yesterday's promises are out the window as soon as your buddy shows up with a six-pack. We might even feel the alcohol coming back up the pipes after a scorching shot of tequila. Maybe we try to convince ourselves, "This is good. Everything is fine. I'm having fun," before swan diving for the nearest upchuck receptacle.

Our cognitive dissonance around alcohol boils down to this: Alcohol is the secret to being cool, attractive, fun, and carefree, and it is an essential part of our cultural and personal identity. But, simultaneously, it is also the ticket to a life of addiction: abuse, job loss, depression, anxiety, DUIs, cancer, brain damage, homelessness, food stamps, and premature death, among many other catastrophic life effects. Because I had yet to connect my conscious mind with my unconscious mind, I was blind to the truth about alcohol. I hadn't yet realized that alcohol was an addictive toxin or that alcohol was a problem. Bill Wilson, the founder of AA, called this his "white light" moment. I call it an awakening. This experience is not some magical, mystical thing that only a few people can make happen. An awakening occurs when you get your unconscious and your conscious mind on the same wavelength. Or, when you can start to wrap your head around your own head. When this happens, the cognitive dissonance reconciles, and you can start to see reality as it is and start making decisions about alcohol, your relationship to it, and your behaviors in accordance with this "white light" realization.

For some, this awakening is a sudden jolt of energy, like the immediate acceptance of a bullshit-free expression of truth. For others, it's much more subtle, a gradual realization that builds slowly over time as you continue to take in information. For me, it was a combination of the two: subtle and slow at first, then all at once. The more I read and studied the scientific research about what alcohol is and what it does to the mind and body, the more I started to ask myself what alcohol had ever really given me. Which put most of my past behavior in a new light. I was starting to realize a few things when I read Annie Grace's groundbreaking book *This Naked Mind*. She says that after reading her book, your mind will be pure, or naked, as it was when you were a child.

By understanding and freeing yourself from the Alcohol Matrix, you will similarly move past the illusion of the collective unconscious and spot, amidst the slowly dissipating cognitive dissonance, conscious reality. The more you observe the scientific truth about alcohol, the more you can resolve your cognitive dissonance and accept the fact that you may in fact have nothing to gain from it. Over the years, I've met a lot of bartenders and winery owners. Very few actually drink. That's not a coincidence. Because they serve alcohol all day, they can't escape reality. They're always watching people waste their money, their time, and their energy. They tell me how quickly that disabuses them of the notion that alcohol is as fun as slogans like "I Don't Get Drunk, I Get Awesome" claim.

The day I was packing up my car before my family's move, I felt great. I was setting out on a new adventure. I thought I knew exactly what I was doing and that I was in total control of my own destiny. As I pulled out of my driveway, I tapped the horn and waved goodbye to Darron, who was still shaking his head. I remember thinking he was in awe, perhaps even a bit jealous, that the normal rules and conventions just didn't apply to me. I was headed toward an exciting new destination, somewhere far away on the horizon, and I had no reason to believe that reality, or its harsh consequences, would ever catch up with me.

I checked the backseat in the rearview mirror and smiled at the case of wine shoehorned between a suitcase and a box of kitchen equipment. When I looked back toward the house, my brother had already started back up the walk. The yard was empty, except for my daughter's car seat, which was still on the blacktop, an image that still haunts me today.

CHAPTER 5

The Lie Alcohol Told Me:
"You're the Most Interesting Man in the World"

The Truth I Figured Out:
Ads for Alcohol Today Are No Different From Ads for Cigarettes Fifty Years Ago

My uncle Gene smoked cigarettes for most of his life. The cigarettes caused cancer in his lungs in the early 1970s. My family and I watched my uncle die in pain, coughing and choking on his own blood. To this day, none of us has ever blamed Gene for dying of lung cancer because we know it was the cigarettes' fault and all of the misinformation about them.

Yet, when esophageal cancer caused by drinking for thirty years killed my dad, we all blamed him. Some members of my family *still* blame my dad for his cancer, even though he hadn't had a drink in more than twenty years by the time he got sick. It wasn't my uncle Gene's fault that he smoked cigarettes and got addicted to them, and they gave him cancer. Nor was it my dad's fault that he got addicted to alcohol, which ultimately gave him cancer. Just like tobacco, alcohol is an addictive, cancer-causing substance. Anyone can get addicted to alcohol, and once they consume enough of it, they *will* get addicted. We must stop blaming the person when it comes to alcohol addiction. And just as my uncle Gene was robbed of half his life by cigarettes, my dad was robbed of his golden years by alcohol because he was programmed throughout his entire life by advertisements that proclaimed alcohol was totally fine, cool, sexy, and fun. His bad behavior was reinforced, if not completely excused, by advertising.

Ad execs continue to follow the same blueprint used to sell cigarettes last century, as portrayed in the *Mad Men* era. It isn't pretty. Nor is it subtle. Nor, as you'll find out, is it anything new! It perpetuates the same misinformation and tired stereotypes about gender that prevented entire generations from living their best lives, including my dad, and continue to try to do the same to me and my generation, and my daughters' generation.

For some of you who skipped the introduction, Annie Grace was the head of global marketing for a large American advertising firm. In 2015 she wrote *This Naked Mind*, the book that enabled me to fully awaken from the illusion of the Alcohol Matrix. Do you think it's a coincidence that it took an advertising specialist to get through to me about my alcohol addiction? Not a psychologist, not a medical doctor, not even a spiritual mentor. Nope. I needed a marketing rep to shake me out of my unconscious slumber. Programming human minds is what Annie was paid to do. In her book, she uses that expertise to deconstruct how advertising is used to get people to drink, explaining how alcohol ads brainwash people, beginning long before they ever have their first drink!

Did you know kids grow up witnessing at least three to four advertisements every single day?[1] In my case, the silly singing cartoon Budweiser frogs and the Spuds McKenzie spotted dog programmed me to associate alcohol with fun. Those ads were not aimed at adults; they were made for kids like me and, as I've since found out, my daughters. I'm astounded when I watch TV with them. There is currently a commercial that keeps popping up for Crown Royal Apple. In the ad, revelers dance to upbeat reggae music in a Caribbean bar as a golden gift from heaven drips sweet apple nectar down on them. The liquid coming out of the apple looks so tasty and fun. All kids know what sugary apple juice tastes like, and I haven't met a kid who doesn't like it. I can see it in my kids' eyes as they watch and wonder to themselves, *Gee, what does that royal apple crown stuff taste like? It looks so fun and yummy!*

Before they have any concept of how awful alcohol really is, the consequences of getting drunk, the addictiveness of alcohol, or the fact that it causes two hundred other diseases and cancers—including the one that killed their grandfather—my two daughters and millions of other kids are drawn in by the incredible marketing. Children watch these types of ads repeatedly as they grow up, and by the time they're teenagers, they're deeply programmed to think alcohol tastes good and is the drink you must have at any adult party.

Advertisements targeted at teens aren't about sweet flavors or funny animals; they're about sex appeal and popularity. Teenagers crave a sense of belonging and appreciation from their peers. Think about the famous, award-winning Dos Equis ad campaign, the perfect ad for people looking to fit in, especially teens and young adults. In the "Most Interesting Man in the World" commercial, a foxy, silver-haired older man is comfortably surrounded by a gaggle of sexy young women. Handsomely clad in a bespoke suit, the Most Interesting Man holds a bottle of Dos Equis. Flashbacks show him as the life of the party, the daring adventurer, the accomplished hero. The ad is basically telling viewers, "If you want to be cool, sexy, and popular for the rest of your life, drink our alcohol." You've probably heard the line: "I don't always drink beer, but when I do . . . I prefer Dos Equis."

"The Most Interesting Man in the World" is one example of sex selling alcohol to teenagers. When I was in high school, I was entranced by the Coors Light girls playing volleyball on the beach, the bikini-clad women shaking their booties against Puff Daddy's tuxedo while he held his vodka for the camera, and the couple making eyes across the room who needed a Johnny Walker to finally make contact. There are an endless number of subliminal messages in alcohol commercials that play to a teenager's hormones and get them riled up and excited to drink. Such messages reinforce gender stereotypes and normalize troubling behavior in both men and women.

TAKE IT FROM BILLY DEE

I remember watching an *In Living Color* sketch lampooning the advertising campaign for Colt 45, a brand of malt liquor. Featuring spokesmodel Billy Dee Williams, the campaign pitched the power of suave sophistication and sexual seduction to audiences, all through malt liquor. This campaign was so egregious that both *Saturday Night Live* and *In Living Color* lampooned its message. Keenen Ivory Wayans, the show's creator and star, portrayed actor Billy Dee Williams, pitching a product called Bolt 45. Dressed in a tuxedo, Wayans sits at the head of a dining room table, surrounded by opulence. "When I'm spending a relaxing evening at home with my very special lady, I like to treat her to the very best," he says into the camera. "I wear the finest clothes, serve the finest gourmet food, and we enjoy the sparkling taste of Bolt 45 malt liquor." His date appears, and Wayans makes a big show of serving her cans of the malt liquor, as if it were a fine wine. He even sniffs the plastic loops the six-pack came in. "Bolt 45 has a fine, rich flavor, a mature multi-bouquet," he continues, while his date chugs can after can. "Bolt

45 also has five times the alcohol content of your average stout beer. So it gets any lady in the mood for what I'm after." Now visibly intoxicated, the date passes out in her chair, and Wayans says, "Somehow I knew she wouldn't refuse me." After putting her on the table, Wayans steps between her legs and delivers the commercial's final pitch. "Remember, if you want class, get champagne. But, if you want to score, get the powerful taste of Bolt 45. Take it from Billy Dee."

The sketch was so controversial, FOX nearly fired Wayans on the spot. Some said it made light of date rape, which it undoubtedly did. But that was kind of the point: the sketch was showing audiences exactly what alcohol advertisements sell, especially to young men. "Alcohol advertisements have effects beyond encouraging people to consume alcohol," says Stacey Hust, a professor at Washington State University's Murrow College of Communication. Hust and her team at the university conducted a study that revealed that alcohol advertising that objectified women encouraged both male and female college students to manipulate others for sex.[2] Both male and female students! Hust and her team showed different alcohol ads to more than one thousand college students—one set of original advertisements featuring highly objectified women, including scantily clad models, and another set of doctored ads featuring the same models wearing a dress, which the study organizers had photoshopped over the original image. The participants then answered questions about the ads, their beliefs in gender stereotypes, sex-related alcohol expectations, and their attitudes toward coercing others into sex with the aid of alcohol. (In the study, sexual coercion covered "a range of negative and illegal behaviors from lying and verbally pressuring someone to plying potential partners with alcohol to have sex.") Male and female subjects who expressed strong beliefs in gender stereotypes, according to Hust and her team, were more likely to sexually coerce, confirming previous research linking gender stereotypes, such as seeing men as sexually aggressive and women as submissive.[3] Although women who expressed a desire to be like the female models in the ads were more likely to use sexual coercion with or without alcohol, this connection was particularly strong with young men who regularly viewed alcohol advertisements that featured objectified female models.

It's not just the message, it's the frequency with which young men find such messages: from billboards and magazines to radio, television, and online, an average of three times a day, or more than one thousand ads per year.[4] Over the past thirty years, advertising firms have successfully placed advertising on programs and in magazines most often seen by young men, especially for hard alcohol. In 1996, producers of spirits put an end to a nearly fifty-year voluntary ban on running ads on radio and television, a kind of gentlemen's agreement in recognition of the social stigma surrounding hard liquor. Once Seagram's aired a commercial for Crown Royal on Prime Sports Network in 1996, the liquor trade association Distilled Spirits Council of the United States, colloquially known as DISCUS, decided to, well, invite every other liquor company to the party.[5] This included Jack Daniel's, Canadian Club, Beefeater, and Smirnoff, among others. One industry insider laid out the new terms. "The members of the distilled-spirits industry have felt for many years that their competitive position has been with one hand tied behind their back," he said, "because they too would like access to a medium they think would be very efficient for them."[6] More efficient than a shot of moonshine, I would say. In 1997, television ads for distilled spirits increased 150 percent: 7,002 ads, in fact.[7] Ads on television jumped to 355 percent the following year, with 12,735 ads appearing on the air.[8] In 2009, more than 14,500 ads for hard liquor aired on television, a 420 percent increase from the end of the ban.[9] Over that time, Nielsen, which counts television viewership, estimates adolescent boys and young between the ages of twelve and twenty saw, on average, 273.6 alcohol ads per year.[10] And, remember, this is only ads on television. A group of underage drinkers watched nearly one ad for alcohol a day! Interestingly, underage youth and drinking-age groups saw more liquor ads than people twenty-five years of age or older.[11]

In 2020, a group at Cornell University examined the effects of such advertising on the drinking habits of young men during this period and beyond, from 2010 to 2013, when the average American saw nearly six hundred ads on television for alcohol per year![12] (It's nearly twice as much across different types of media.) "These ads are so ubiquitous, especially for certain types of audiences, that this cumulative, repeated exposure seems to have the potential to reinforce the behavior," said Jeff Niederdeppe, associate professor of communication at the College of Agriculture and Life Sciences at Cornell, in a press release about his study. "Higher exposure to the ads is clearly and consistently linked to higher levels of drinking." He and his team estimated that "a doubling of exposure to alcohol ads would increase by 11 percent the odds that someone reported having at least one drink in the last 30 days, and among drinkers would increase by 5 percent the number of drinks consumed during the previous month."[13] (African Americans saw about 150 more commercials a year than white survey respondents, according to Niederdeppe.[14])

"Maybe it's a handful of drinks, but it's a handful of drinks spread across a very large number of people," Niederdeppe said. "To the extent that increases in alcohol consumption, particularly at high levels, are associated with negative health outcomes, then there's the potential for a significant effect at the population level. It makes clear that there's a huge volume of exposure that is potentially consequential."

Potentially consequential? That's a bit of an understatement, don't you think? The consequence of alcohol's increasing ubiquity within our culture only strengthens its cultural power and our unconscious connection to it, in much the same way as tobacco once did. Comparing tobacco's influence to alcohol's might today seem like we're comparing an ant to dragon. But smoking used to be a major part of our culture, a fire-spitting-and-smoke-breathing dragon of yesteryear that was an essential part of our collective identity, only slightly behind religion, baseball, and apple pie. However, as we saw with cigarettes, it's entirely possible to take down cultural dragons and shift away from lies and influence. An anti-smoking reform movement began in the 1880s because of concerns over the hygienic standards of cigarettes. To dissolve these concerns, a milder tobacco blend was developed in the early twentieth century that made the smoke easier to inhale, therefore increasing nicotine absorption into the bloodstream. During World War I, surgeons endorsed cigarettes for their sedative-like effects on wounded soldiers. When cigarettes went into mass production, they were seen as cool, sexy, mature, tasty, and even healthy. Doctors would smoke cigarettes in their exam rooms, and Big Tobacco marketers conditioned people to think that life would be so much better with a smoke in hand. The old cigarette commercials showed gorgeous models smoking in limousines with a bottle of champagne nearby. If you were a soldier fighting for your country and didn't smoke, there was something wrong with you. Tobacco use was ubiquitous in the media and in social circles. However, when scientific research made the indisputable claim that cigarettes led to a whole host of health problems, including arthritis, diabetes, and cancer, it didn't take long for the so-called benefits of cigarettes to fall out of fashion.

SMOKING BANS BEGIN

Tobacco's downfall started in the middle of the century. In the 1950s, lung cancer cases sharply increased, becoming the most prevalent cancer among American males. It was apparent that the widespread popularity of cigarette smoking was linked to this increase in cancer. By the 1960s, anti-smoking campaigns caused cigarette sales to dramatically decrease, as anyone who's ever watched *Mad Men* can tell you. During the 1970s, probably around the same time Don Draper was—spoiler alert!—dreaming up his famous ad for Coca-Cola, the US government banned smoking in government facilities, including the Armed Forces! Throughout the 1990s, Big Tobacco paid hundreds of millions of dollars in legal settlements for tobacco-related illnesses in the United States. By 1999, advertisements for Big Tobacco were almost entirely restricted, and cigarette companies were required to spend $100 million toward anti-tobacco advertisements.

In the span of about a century, the United States introduced, popularized, debunked, and dethroned cigarettes. Today, most societies are up front about the dangers associated with cigarettes. Cigarette packages throughout Europe are plastered with horrifying images of holes in people's throats, birth defects, mouths with no lips, and black lungs. They are not portrayed as healthy or necessary. We are aghast at the doctors who endorsed smoking.

Sadly, under our current political system, alcohol commercials have no obligation to discuss alcohol-related disease, short- or long-term effects of alcohol consumption, or the addictive properties of alcohol. They lie to us and our children about what alcohol actually does, simply because they can. There are no legal ramifications whatsoever. These blatant lies and lack of information feed the Alcohol Matrix and contribute to an insane culture that celebrates drinking an addictive substance but disgraces those who've become addicted to it.

In 1988, the Alcoholic Beverage Labeling Act required all alcoholic beverages to include health warning labels on their bottles and packaging. The only risks deemed necessary to include, however, were the following: (1) according to the Surgeon General, women should not drink alcoholic beverages during pregnancy because of the risk of birth defects; and (2) the consumption of alcoholic beverages impairs your ability to drive a car or operate machinery and may cause health problems.

Despite a long history of alcohol addiction and abuse in the United States, many lawmakers believed (and were paid by Big Alcohol lobbyists to believe) that the science at the time was "inconclusive" and didn't necessarily prove that alcohol led to cancer, disease, and abusive behaviors. Well, lawmakers of today, the science *is* conclusive. Still, Big Alcohol lobbyists continue to distort scientific research in their favor to avoid responsibility for alcohol-related deaths and growing rates of addiction in America. Big Alcohol invests millions into campaigns that promote the idea that drinking is good for you and can even benefit your health, from Michelob's USDA-certified organic mango apricot seltzer that is gluten-free and six times filtered with zero grams of added sugar to White Claw's ridiculous claim that their hard sparkling water, aimed at weight-obsessed college students and fitness-conscious moms, contains only a hundred calories. Modelo beer put out quite the ad for the Olympics, featuring swimmer Nathan Adrian, an eight-time Olympic medalist and cancer survivor. The ad says he is a lion for his fortitude in continuing to train despite such a great obstacle. It then shows Nathan smiling and sitting around a campfire with friends, about to drink alcohol—which is proven to cause cancer. The tagline? "Modelo: brewed for those with a fighting spirit." I am not saying that Nathan Adrian got cancer just from drinking alcohol. What I *am* saying is that this is one of the most blatant attempts by Big Alcohol to cover up the facts.

As the world starts to figure out how alcohol advertising purposely distorts reality and perpetuates the Alcohol Matrix, ad execs are trying to integrate alcohol into our everyday lives in more deliberate ways, aligning alcoholic products with notable charitable causes and specific groups. A handful of alcohol campaigns claim to be doing the world a favor by donating to charities and raising awareness for problems such as domestic violence and cancer. This is a practice known as "charity washing." One prominent example of this type of campaign has been dubbed "pinkwashing" by critics. This refers to Big Alcohol putting a pink ribbon around their products to help raise awareness for those fighting breast cancer. This is extremely callous and hypocritical advertising, because the fact is that thousands of breast cancer cases are *caused* by the consumption of alcohol. As breastcancer.org notes, "Compared to women who don't drink at all, women who have three alcoholic drinks per week have a 15 percent higher risk of breast cancer. Experts estimate that the risk of breast cancer goes up another 10 percent for each additional drink women regularly have each day."[15] The American Cancer Society notes that alcohol consumption is the "third-highest cause of cancer, after cigarette smoking and excessive body weight."[16]

If Big Alcohol really cared about improving women's health, they would put bright yellow cancer warnings on the bottles instead of pink ribbons. This hypocrisy can also be found in Big Alcohol giving money to charities for rehabilitating the homeless, who are often without a place to live because of an addiction to alcohol. The same can be said about supporting charities that work with victims of domestic abuse. The World Health Organization (WHO) estimates that roughly 55 percent of domestic abuse perpetrators were drinking alcohol prior to committing assault.[17] The New York State Office for the Prevention of Domestic Violence, meanwhile, reports that violence against female partners was two to four times more common in men with alcohol problems than among other men, and abusive men who binge drink or take illicit drugs were more likely to have an increased risk of their violent behavior resulting in the death of their partners.[18] More than 80 percent of men who abused or killed female partners were problem drinkers in the year preceding the incident, and more than two-thirds of men who tried to kill or killed their partners were drunk at the time of the incident.[19]

We're so programmed, we think alcohol brands sponsoring charity is a good thing instead of realizing they're trying to cover up their wrongs. I'm not saying it's bad for Big Alcohol to give a tiny portion of their money to a worthy cause. However, it is important to recognize the complete hypocrisy of these actions and see that Big Alcohol could be doing a lot more to prevent cancer, abuse, drunk driving deaths, and fetal alcohol syndrome at the source instead of paying reparations. Does this remind anyone of Big Tobacco? Does it make you shiver a little when you hear about the Philip Morris–funded "Foundation for a Smoke-Free World," when they are now trying to push their highly addictive, nicotine smoke–free vape products instead of cigarettes? That gives a whole new meaning to the word *smokescreen*!

Years ago, I met my dad one afternoon for lunch. He was seventy-four and hadn't had a drink in twenty years. He had finished his daily three-mile run, which he completed religiously. He and I both ordered the grilled salmon. While we ate, I noticed he was having trouble swallowing his bites. The next afternoon, barely twenty-four hours later, my dad went to the doctor, who diagnosed him with the esophageal cancer that would kill him six months later, the same cancer he developed after years of alcohol abuse.

In the time between my lunch with my dad and his terminal diagnosis, the average American adolescent and adult was exposed to five to ten ads for alcohol either on television, magazine ads, billboards, or radio spots, and the average American kid watched at least three in between their favorite TV shows. Now, whenever I see an advertisement for alcohol, I say my adapted version of the line from *The Princess Bride*: "HELLO! My name is Dustin Dunbar! You killed my father. Prepare to die!"

But let me be clear: I am not saying that we should ban cigarettes or alcohol. I am a free will–loving American who doesn't like to be told what I can and cannot do. And we're all aware of the damage and civic disruption Prohibition caused the nation. We should all be able to make our own choices with tobacco and alcohol. But now that we know for a fact that alcohol causes cancer and two hundred other diseases, and that it is addictive to anyone who consumes enough of it, we must put updated warning labels on bottles and cans that contain alcohol, just like we do on cigarette packs. And we need to ban alcohol ads the same way we ban cigarette ads. All of us, especially our children, should not be inundated with daily lies about how fun, sexy, and even healthy it is to drink an addictive, cancer-causing poison. This is not difficult. More than fifty years ago, we banned cigarettes ads. In 1970, Congress passed the Public Health Cigarette Smoking Act, banning the advertising of cigarettes on television and radio. It is time we do the same for alcohol. Stop all of the brainwashing. Stop all the misinformation. Stop the lies. Big Alcohol has made enough money using our bodies and brains to feed the Alcohol Matrix.

I like to get detailed when I imagine things happening in the future because we create what we imagine and strive to achieve.

Which is why I make a practice of looking forward to the headline, "Congress Passes the Public Health Alcohol Act, Banning the Advertising of Alcohol Starting on January 12, 2028."

I recently read a Bloomberg article with the headline, "Florida in $879 Million Opioid Settlement With CVS, Allergan and Teva." In the body of the article, was this paragraph: "The suits seek compensation for billions of tax dollars spent battling the opioid epidemic, which has claimed more than 500,000 lives in the U.S. over the past 20 years. U.S. states, cities and counties have recovered more than $32 billion so far to beef up budgets for police, drug-treatment and other social-service needs."[20]

Imagine the suits seeking compensation for Big Alcohol's role in three million global deaths per year. Modelo better have their "fighting spirit" and tons of money ready, because just like Big Tobacco and opioid pharmaceutical companies had to pay billions of dollars in legal fees, so too will Modelo and every company that continues to put ads for alcohol in front of us and our children.

DETOX TIMELINE: ONE MONTH ALCOHOL-FREE

A month in was when my mind really started feeling clear. My body was clean. I dropped ten pounds, really without changing much other than eliminating alcohol. I was still deep into my research and practicing repetition and visualization. I was getting better at communicating my thoughts and my feelings—and articulating my personal boundaries. In fact, I told my ex-wife about a month in that I wasn't going to drink with her ever again. I told my drinking brothers the same thing. I was clear and confident, thanks in no small part to the repetition and visualization exercise I'd practiced in my first month alcohol-free.

This is when I realized that this wasn't a so-called dry period; it was a permanent lifestyle change. And this is when you start figuring out how to actualize this change into every part of your life.

I am a Green Bay Packers fan because the team is owned by the people instead of a single billionaire who can just move away when they choose. Vince Lombardi, who coached the Packers, is such an influential figure in football history that the Super Bowl trophy is named after him.. He had a signature recipe for success that I know from firsthand experience also works for beating alcohol addiction. Vince's key to leading numerous teams to championships was a repetition of the fundamental elements of the sport. He would start off every season by going back to the absolute basics. On the first day of practice, he would hold up a football for the team and coaching staff to see, and say, "This is a football." Then he would recite the rules and history of the sport to remind his team of the truths of football and to renew their understanding and love of the game. He didn't take anything for granted and believed that even top athletes and high-end professionals need to be reminded of the basics every year.

Just like Lombardi, we must continually remind ourselves and our children of the truth about alcohol. We must keep our minds and our children's minds clean from the lies of the unconscious Alcohol Matrix and Big Alcohol advertising. When you watch or hear an ad about alcohol with your children, tell them some scientific facts about the dangers of alcohol while the ad plays. You will be amazed by how many times you must do this each day if you do it each time one comes on! It's exhausting, but it always feels right.

When it is active, alcohol addiction lives inside of you. It literally takes over your mind and body. It becomes an incessantly powerful voice in your head. "You earned a drink. Just one. Take it easy and relax." If you listen to this addict voice or do not pay close attention to your addiction, you will see yourself with a drink in your hand and not even realize how it got there because of years with this compulsive habit. One of my favorite authors, Eckhart Tolle, advises that when compulsive needs arise, you can stop and take three breaths. Doing this generates awareness and allows you to recognize the urge for what it is.

This practice worked for me. And I know it will work for you. The next time you feel the need to drink, notice the thoughts that try to justify your addiction.

Maybe just one small glass of wine tonight.

It's a bachelor party; I can let loose.

All of my friends will be there.

This is your addiction talking. Breathe. Be the witness of your addict thoughts. If you become present and aware of this addict voice, it will have no power over you.

If you want to remain alcohol-free for life, you must have the deep conviction in the depths of your being, both consciously and subconsciously, that alcohol is a toxic substance and you are disgusted by it, just like an old cigarette addict is disgusted by smoking today. To train the subconscious, remind yourself of the facts whenever you're around the stuff. Recall how it harmed you, how it will harm you again, and that you don't want to be harmed. Remember how it has harmed your family and friends. Cravings can only occur when we perceive a benefit. Get your conscious and subconscious in alignment with the truth, and you'll see alcohol for what it is: a poison.

By getting this far, you've proven you're serious about cutting poison from your life, and this can speak volumes to your loved ones, colleagues, and employers. This might be a good time to talk to loved ones about your alcohol addiction. It is incredibly healthy to share your thoughts and feelings with people who are important to you. Go through your personal list of people and really consider if they are true loved ones and friends, or if they were just drinking buddies.

Remember to apologize deeply to those you hurt with your drinking. The length of time it takes to address interpersonal harm varies by person and situation. A genuine apology can help mend and strengthen injured relationships as you move forward in whatever new form the relationship takes. Also remember to say sorry to the kids and teens in your life. I can assure you that if you drank for any amount of time around your kids, you need to apologize to them. Remember, you are trying to model good behavior. Make sure they really hear your apology. This is an opportunity to show them that all people make mistakes. Your apology shows them how to be vulnerable and take responsibility. They need to know that when they make mistakes, they can come to you with their problems and not hide them or feel ashamed of them. Apologize and then share your plan to stay healthy and present in their lives. Listen to what they have to say about your plan. Kids can be great cheerleaders. You can use their encouragement and faith in you to strengthen your resolve.

PART III

THE HEAD,
THE HEART,
AND THE SOUL

CHAPTER 6

The Lie Alcohol Told Me:
"Alcohol Takes the Edge Off"

The Truth I Figured Out:
Alcohol *Is* the Edge

Because of what I shared about my dad, you'll probably find it hard to believe that he didn't really drink until he was in his midtwenties. He was already married and a father of three. Once he started drinking, though, he couldn't stop. His descent into addiction was quick. A beer to unwind after work quickly became three or four, which then turned into a bottle of vodka. Like most other drinkers, my dad fell victim to the lie that he needed a drink because alcohol "takes the edge off."

Growing up, I came to fear that saying because he said it right before things broke bad.

My dad was addicted to alcohol. He was also a narcissist. He grew up without any love, validation, or even attention from my grandparents. Despite his good looks and high intelligence, my father suffered from low self-esteem. Because he had been deprived of love and attention as a child, he craved them both as an adult, and he came to believe, as many people do—me included—that alcohol helps you get both. This doesn't excuse his behavior, but it helps explain it. As a father, he repeated his parents' behavior, conscious and unconscious alike, and treated his love first as a gift and then as a weapon. Affection and anger were one and the same, or at least different sides of the same coin, and we never really knew on which side he was going to land. I'm not sure my dad knew either. I now believe he relied on alcohol to make the decision for him. For him, "taking the edge off" was an attempt to stay even-keeled. But it was more Russian roulette, a random chance, than an effective relaxation technique.

Regardless of his mood, whenever my dad drank, he wasn't present with his family. He was there, but he wasn't present. He was awake, but he was acting unconsciously. He was the alcohol-induced monster who dragged my mom out of the house by her hair more times than I'd like to admit. Alcohol hadn't taken the edge off on that morning, or any other morning, or any other day. At that moment, and during many other moments throughout his life, alcohol had taken him over completely.

As I got older and continued to drink more alcohol, my tolerance increased—so I drank more. I would bargain with myself, and I could always come up with excuses to drink, even though I knew it was hurting me in the short and long term. If it were a special occasion, for instance, my immediate reaction was to hit the boutique wine store to stock up. If I were going out, I needed to make drinks . . . to get ready to go out and drink. Pregaming, we proudly call it. If there was a big sporting event, I would have everyone over in the morning for a fully stocked Bloody Mary bar, followed by lots of beers during the game and drinks post-game. If I was on vacation, I scheduled my itinerary around wine tastings, champagne brunches, brewery tours, happy hours, and craft brew pubs. I found every socially acceptable excuse to have more addictive poison. And just like every person who has ever been addicted, including my dad, I was in full denial and couldn't see my alcohol addiction. I was on Alcohol Matrix–induced autopilot, hardly making any conscious decisions other than finding another reason to have another drink.

Throughout this period, my mood was on a steep decline. I gained twenty extra pounds of fat. Surfing was no longer as much fun because I didn't have the strength or the stamina. Of course, I didn't want to give up the alcohol I was addicted to, so I compensated for my declining health with more exercise and dieting. I worked out for an hour a day, telling myself later that evening that I'd earned a drink. However, the alcohol affected me more intensely each month, and my love of exercise turned into a painful chore as decreased energy levels made every activity twice as painful and difficult. When I was living in Thailand in my late thirties, I tried Buddhist meditation again, a practice I first fell in love with when I was in graduate school. Back then, I would take an hour-long meditation class every day, sometimes twice a day. My fateful drink in Milan put an end to that, unfortunately. But if I thought it was hard to exercise with a hangover, I learned in Thailand that exercise was a proverbial walk in the park compared with trying to stay in the present moment! The problem was, I couldn't stay awake during meditations because I was red-eyed and weary from the previous night's drinking: four bottles of 4.8 percent alcohol Chang beer, and a nightcap glass of 13 percent alcohol red wine, a brutal cocktail that yielded little more than low energy levels, a cloudy brain, an achy body, and an anxious spirit. It was no wonder I couldn't make it through meditation without passing out. Looking back, I recognize the irony of sleeping through the same kind of meditation exercises I love so much today. It's safe to say I was pretty much sleeping through everything else, even if I was awake. That's my definition of a living nightmare.

While I was sleepwalking through life, Darron was living his own nightmare. He was waking up after a long night of drinking

and dry-heaving most of the day until he had to go to work waiting tables. He'd work until 10 p.m., then go straight to a bar,
where he stayed most of the night. One day, one of his friends,
the most famous drag queen in San Francisco, saw Darron walking around the neighborhood. Suffering from what he described
as "a particularly horrific hangover," he was wearing a pair of
dirty jeans and a T-shirt, en route to getting a huge Dr Pepper
and two of the greasiest slices of pepperoni pizza he could find.

When his friend saw him, he said, "Gurl, you look a wreck!
What is going on?"

"Oh, it's the drinking every night. I'm just so sick all the time."

"Oh, gurl, I remember all that. It was so bad I'd have to wake up
and have a drink to stop the dry heaves and get through the day,
and that made me just a full-time, sloppy-ass drunk. I couldn't
keep a job, no one wanted to be around me, I'd make a fool out
of myself onstage; until one day a friend of mine drug me to a
meeting and I stopped drinking. And thank God. I was so gross
and unhappy and probably close to death. Quitting drinking
saved my life. If you ever wanna go, call me and I'll meet you
there, cause oof, gurl, you look pretty close to death yourself."

What part of that story do you think Darron heard? Not the
offer to help him quit drinking. No, what Darron heard was the
idea that he could just start drinking as soon as he woke up. The
next morning, after another long night of drinking, he woke
up, puked, went to the fridge, and downed a huge tumbler of
white Zinfandel. "That gut-wringing, dry-heaving hangover was
replaced with a numb bubble that made the world look like I had
Vaseline on my eyes," he later told me. "All those nagging feelings
of responsibility and not throwing my life away and cleaning up
my damn room once in a while just magically went away."

Darron kept up like that until his roommate and our cousin
confronted him. "Something gotta give," they said, before

shipping him back to Oklahoma for his first thirty-day stint in rehab.

OPERANT CONDITIONING

Unless you're a character from a TV show or beer commercial, you probably know that alcohol produces negative effects, like hangovers and disorientation. However, if you're like 84 percent of adult Americans, you will drink at some point in your lifetime.[1] So why doesn't your awareness of the consequences condition you to *avoid* drinking? Why haven't you developed a Pavlovian association between taking a tequila shot and vomiting in the sink? The problem is that there's another, more powerful form of conditioning at work that overpowers the Pavlovian kind. Championed by psychologist B. F. Skinner in the 1930s, *operant conditioning* is a real powerhouse within the Alcohol Matrix. Operant conditioning comes down to two simple concepts: reward and punishment.[2] When you perceive rewards for drinking alcohol, you'll feel the desire to go out drinking again. When you are punished for drinking, you'll be deterred. The problem is, you have been conditioned your entire life to view alcohol as rewarding. So what if you slur your speech or can't stand up straight? So what if you forget who you slept with after that New Year's Eve party? These types of negative associations and minor punishments are a drop in the bucket compared with the rewards we have been conditioned to perceive—especially when the Alcohol Matrix twists those punishments into social rewards the next day, when you and your buddies laugh and bond over your hangover stories and blackout moments. Then, eventually, you remind yourself that you need a drink and start up again—a little hair of the dog, of course, to help take the edge off.

Look, I get it. I do. Why wouldn't you believe this? Like me, and my dad, and Darron, you were taught to believe that alcohol takes the edge off.

Well, it doesn't. It never has. And it never will.

Alcohol can't help take the edge off because alcohol *is* the edge. It's the primary source of stress!

Rather than taking the edge off, alcohol increases your heart rate and your blood pressure. Your body has to work harder to break it down and purge the poisonous effects of alcohol from your bloodstream. And, as I'm sure you already know, increased heart rate and blood pressure often lead to increased levels of stress. To make matters worse, alcohol's deadening effects attenuate with tolerance, so drinkers end up consuming more poison and experiencing more side effects to reach a desired numbing effect. That's exactly what happened to me.

Alcohol also causes physiological changes in your brain. When you're drinking, there's an influx of gamma aminobutyric acid (GABA) that causes you to feel relaxed and calm. As soon as you stop drinking, you immediately start to experience symptoms of withdrawal, which spikes stress levels and incites deep feelings of anxiety. Dr. Carl Erik Fisher, an addiction psychiatrist at Columbia University, explained in an article in the *New York Times* that "it really causes profound physical effects across a variety of different systems." Alcohol "affects the kidneys, immune system, brain, hormones, metabolism and the circulatory system," among other things.[3]

It's no wonder why hangovers are so tough. It's not just the dehydration! Our bodies are trying to recalibrate and reset, all while trying to purge our system of alcohol's poison. As bad as hangovers are, they're exacerbated twofold by something we've casually come to term "hangxiety," a feeling of being worn out both mentally and physically and a bit shaky emotionally. It's amazing how clever we can all be when we want to make light of something we all know is terrible for us. Wine o'clock, Sunday Funday, pregaming, hair of the dog, take the edge off. They all sound so quaint, so homespun. There's no way they could hint at anything so deleterious or self-destructive. But they do. Think about what it feels like to experience hangxiety. You're listless and exhausted. Jittery and depressed. You're on edge, shaky, and most likely sweaty. Now think about what it feels like to suffer from alcohol withdrawal. You're listless and exhausted. Jittery and depressed. You're on edge, shaky, and most likely sweaty. This is not a coincidence. For people who drink to excess, hangxiety can last for days or weeks or even months. This is called post-acute alcohol withdrawal syndrome, or PAWS, another cute acronym. But at least this one communicates the negative effects alcohol has on us.

As recent studies on diabetes show, drinking causes our stress hormones to increase, and our blood sugar can become either too low or too high, which is why we experience hangxiety.[4] When we're hungover, our brain experiences changes that make it difficult to regulate anxiety. Studies show that people who already suffer with mood disorders are more likely to experience hangxiety. Any additional stress—including drinking alcohol—can exacerbate the physiological effects of specific disorders. What's more, new research has also revealed that shy people are prone to suffer with hangxiety, which supports the link between social anxiety and alcohol abuse that we referenced in Chapter 2.

Another symptom of hangxiety is interrupted sleep, which compounds feelings of depression and anxiety. In a 2022 study, researchers served one volunteer group alcoholic drinks—men had approximately five and women had four—and served another group mocktails throughout the evening.[5] Researchers then monitored the volunteers' sleep activity through the night. They found that alcohol consumption reduced both the total amount of time the subjects slept and the amount of time they spent in REM sleep compared with those who didn't drink alcohol. Commenting on the study in the *New York Times*, our addiction specialist Dr. Fisher put it this way: "Your sleep quality is just not as good, even though the number of hours you're spending unconscious may be the same."

You know what I love most about Dr. Fisher's quote? The fact that he purposely used the word *unconscious*. Though I dive deep into this subject later, I do want to point out here how none of us are ever fully conscious during addiction, when we're still stuck firmly in the Alcohol Matrix. You aren't. My dad wasn't. Darron wasn't. And I certainly wasn't.

Kicking your addiction to alcohol is the only way to start feeling better about yourself and finally figure out how to navigate the kind of stressful and hectic moments life inevitably throws your way.

Fear and anxiety are ever-present forces in most people's lives. Unfortunately, most of us aren't trained to confront this fear and get to the root of it. That's why many people turn to alcohol. Instead of confronting our fears and anxieties, we go through life drunk and unable to realize that there are ways to de-stress that *don't* require poisoning our minds and bodies. Even though we know that alcohol is harmful to our bodies, we are too afraid to experience life without the comfort we've associated with alcohol for so long. The Alcohol Matrix allows us to be numb and unconscious.

We're stuck in a deadly cycle where stress and alcohol feed off each other. This cycle makes us blind to the possibility of relaxation in regular, alcohol-free life. Alcohol doesn't make us better at handling stress. It just makes us less aware. Your stress hasn't magically disappeared; it will always be there regardless of how much you try to avoid it. If you continue using alcohol to suppress your fears, you'll never truly overcome them, and you will suffer more in the end.

To keep living in this deadly cycle of pain, you can keep drinking. But if you want to stop relying on a substance to (ineffectively) duck your problems, end the cycle by experiencing life fully alcohol-free. Give yourself permission to face your fears and anxieties without repressing them. Stop using alcohol to stifle your brain activity. Use 100 percent of your conscious mind, 100 percent of the time, and train yourself to handle stress as it comes. Once you stop turning to the bottle for stress relief, you'll be able to fully investigate the real sources of stress and fear.

Experiencing the full spectrum of your emotions doesn't have to be gloom and doom all the time. Anxiety isn't the only emotion that gets out of whack in the presence of ethanol. Joy can be stifled by alcohol, too.

FROM THE HEART

Here's another story, one with a happy ending. I promise.

After about a year of being separated from my ex-wife and only seeing my girls half the time, I felt a severe dull pain in my chest, right where my heart is. It got so bad that I went to the ER, where I had all kinds of tests. Doctors told me everything checked out fine, that it was probably pleurisy, or lung inflammation, the result of overexercising.

"No," I kept telling them, "it is not my lung. I can feel exactly where it is. It's inside my heart."

I went to a lung specialist, who ordered more tests. Her scan of my chest showed an aortic root aneurysm. I went to a cardiologist, who said the aneurysm was large enough that I would need to have open-heart surgery. I was in complete shock. The cardiologist told me that the root of the aorta is where the aorta connects to the heart, not the long part of the aorta that's a simple tube. This meant the surgery would be much more difficult than putting a stent in. I was told that some do not survive the surgery, and the ones that do have a much lower life expectancy afterward.

After my cardiologist went through my health history, he couldn't understand how or why I got this aneurysm at my young age. He said my physical condition was too good and my family tree didn't have any heart problems.

I told him what you already know: as a child I was psychologically abused and abandoned by my father. Because of this, throughout my life, I had an extremely unconscious fear of being abandoned. I spent my life trying to get love and validation from everyone and everything. Then my wife, whom I love so much, asked to be separated, and the extremely unconscious fear of being abandoned by my family was so bad that it put me in a mental health treatment center for a month. There I became conscious of my fear and found out that it is formally called love addiction. The symptoms I showed were extreme anxiety, fear, and depression. I told him all this because I knew that the aneurysm was psychosomatic and that my unconscious mind caused my broken heart.

Because of Covid, it took another two months to get more detailed scans on my aortic root, and they came out much better than previously thought. Thankfully, the aneurysm is currently not large enough to have to operate. But for the two months that I thought I was going to undergo extreme open-heart surgery, I faced all anxiety and fear of death head-on. I didn't drink a drop of alcohol. I didn't take any drugs. I was completely alcohol-free. And you know what happened? I quieted my anxiety and, in the process, started to find joy. I never needed surgery, and I still feel great today.

You might wonder what you'll turn to without alcohol around

to keep your anxiety low. I relied on exercise and meditation. Yoga and sleep, too. These were my favorite ways to take the edge off. And, unlike alcohol, they didn't leave me hungover or anxious or ashamed about my behavior. They also didn't make me miss drinking. They empowered me to know and say out loud that I didn't need alcohol for any reason. At all.

Exercise calmed my mind, rebuilt my muscles, and reconditioned my cardiovascular system. Exercise will give you better pastimes than hanging out at the bar or watching TV with a beer in your hand. Even better, you can make new friends at your classes while getting in shape and sweating out any leftover toxins.

Meditation was my favorite tool in my recovery. It was also the most powerful. Meditation is linked to a variety of health benefits, including managing anxiety, stress, depression, pain, and symptoms related to withdrawal from nicotine, alcohol, or opioids.[6] Additionally, training your mind to witness your thoughts allows you to break the lies you've accepted over the years. Meditation is your Get Out of Jail Free card. Or, I guess I should say, your Get Out of the Alcohol Matrix Free card.

If you haven't done so already, start a daily meditation practice. Through meditation, you'll be able to gain new clarity to tackle any obstacle life throws at you. The best advice I have ever received about meditation is to "keep starting over." Even the greatest Zen masters get their thoughts hijacked while meditating. Starting over is simply bringing your full attention back to your breath. You can focus where your breath flows—in and out of your nose—or you can focus on your belly or chest rising and falling. That's it. The more you start over, the more time will pass before you start over again. Your ego and thinking mind will try to tell you that nothing is happening, and that meditation is boring and ineffective. You may not notice anything while meditating; where you will notice a difference is in your daily life. After you have meditated for about a month, start asking yourself: Am I more at peace than I was before meditating daily? Do I seem to have more compassion for others after a month of meditation? If you focus on your breath, or a single point like a candle flame or your third eye, every day for a month, I can tell you the odds are very good that you will feel more peaceful and compassionate.

Be kind to yourself when you realize you are thinking during meditation. No need to get upset or frustrated at all. I used to beat myself up for getting hijacked by a thought. Now I just come back gently with the voice of Jeff Spicoli, the surfer from the classic movie *Fast Times at Ridgemont High*. I think to myself in Spicoli's voice, *Whoa . . . dude. Paddle back into your breath bro, you're thinking. That's better. Now stay completely still, chill, and ride the tasty wave of no-thought.*

Yoga is an incredible way to bring your body, mind, and spirit together as one. Your entire being will leave your session feeling cleansed from the inside out with a peaceful rejuvenation. It reminds me of the feeling I have after a full-body massage, which is about as good as it gets. I highly recommend mixing in sessions of yoga anytime you can.

"Sleep is the best meditation," the Dalai Lama tells us. Since I have been alcohol-free, the amount of sleep I need goes in waves. Some nights I will only sleep five hours and wake up as fresh as ever, and some nights I go to bed early and sleep ten hours because my mind and body are telling me that's what I need. Sleep keeps us calm, lowers blood pressure, and has tons of other major health benefits. Never feel guilty if your mind or body wants to sleep. Almost daily in the afternoon, I do a quick twenty-minute savasana sleep meditation, also known as a nap. Usually between 1 p.m. and 4 p.m., our circadian rhythm (biological sleep clock) drops down and naturally makes us feel drowsy.

Historically, scientists believe this was when humans needed to get out of the midday sun. I don't fight against this rhythm with energy drinks and/or caffeine anymore. If I have to, I lean the seat of my car all the way back and take a quick nap that way.

Once you get past the initial struggle to quit drinking and escape the Alcohol Matrix, you'll bask in the white light that comes with experiencing an alcohol awakening. You'll feel empowered by the consciousness high that comes with being alcohol-free, and you'll be thankful you never have to experience the negative side effects of alcohol again. You'll be free to discover all the personal growth that alcohol has stunted for so many years, and you'll enjoy life more fully. No more lagging on your daily exercise because your damaged organs make you fatigued. No more popping pills after a night of drinking to kill the pain. No more regrets over the hurtful things you said or did when you were drunk.

It's not a new you; it's who you were all along and were always meant to be.

My third month living alcohol-free occurred in the middle of the holiday season. December 19 was exactly three months from that last Bloody Mary. I have to admit it was an odd time. I had just gone through twenty-eight years of drinking through the holidays, then suddenly not. Everywhere I went, I saw alcohol. The stores were stocked with liquor and beer. I received bottles of wine as gifts. I went to one Christmas party after another.

And I felt great. Joy and lightness were coming out of me.

Thanks to my steady protocol of research, repetition, visualization (plus exercise and mediation, of course), I could recognize the Alcohol Matrix in full effect. I could also see that it no longer had any effect on me.

I must admit, though, that I was lonely, primarily because I was the only person in my life who wasn't drinking alcohol. I remember leaning into my incredibly supportive online community on the I Am Sober app, which helped a great deal. Another thing that helped me was listening more to people who had already awakened from the Alcohol Matrix. People like Annie Grace, my Morpheus (a character in the movie *The Matrix*). I listened to the audio version of her book so many times in between Thanksgiving and Christmas. No matter how many times I finished the recording, I always came away refreshed and inspired, fully awake. I always knew that, like Neo (from *The Matrix*), I had a choice: I could go back to sleep or wake up and be conscious.

After three months, you've probably encountered a holiday, anniversary, or celebration of some kind. These can be challenging moments for the newly awakened and alcohol-free. It can feel strange to enter a social situation where your unconscious is programmed to drink. This is where the kind of visualization exercises I discussed previously really pay off. Prior to going to a party, visualize yourself there and activate your senses. What do you hear? What do you smell? Who's there? What do you want to say?

Some drinkers at a given event won't be fully aware of and fully receptive to your newfound freedom and will offer you drinks. Some will find it odd that you're not partaking. In these situations, even as an adult, you may be heavily peer pressured to drink. However, the Alcohol Matrix speaking through your peers doesn't have a chance with you anymore. You are awake now, and conscious of its every ploy. This is a period when some alcohol-free people become self-assured and begin to realize they can overcome any temptation.

Notice any collective unconscious falsehoods that pop into your head, like, "It will be fine to have just one." You know the problem isn't the amount. You are still dealing with the same addictive poison. One drink quickly turns into two, and then back to more frequent use, escalating fast.

Years of drinking have not been erased from our minds, nor will they ever be. If we start drinking again, we pick back up again where we left off drinking, not at square one. Our brains remember exactly where we stopped drinking, which was in some stage of addiction. Remember that making the drinkers around you more comfortable with their own addiction is not worth going back to being addicted and putting poisonous car fuel in your body and mind.

Achieving alcohol-free harmony between your conscious and unconscious requires regular practice. It's like learning a second language. Learning Spanish in middle school doesn't mean you will be able to hold a fluent conversation for the rest of your life.

You will still be bombarded by Big Alcohol advertisements telling your subconscious how wonderful alcohol is. To continue to see through the Alcohol Matrix and Big Alcohol lies and stay alcohol-free for life, you need to constantly remind yourself of the truth about alcohol. The Alcohol Matrix and Big Alcohol are both relentless, so you need to be relentless as well in constantly feeding your mind the scientific truth that alcohol is an addictive, cancer-causing poison. One trick I still like to use is to turn around every alcohol advertisement I see, stating scientific truths for every false benefit that I encounter about alcohol. For example, a Coors Light ad says, "Taste the Rockies: Uniquely Crisp, Refreshing, Drinkable." I say, "Taste the Ethanol: Uniquely Toxic, Dehydrating, Deadening." This utilizes the power of operant conditioning by highlighting the punishments associated with alcohol and downplaying the proposed rewards. This technique will always outwit and outmatch Big Alcohol's attempts to program you.

CHAPTER 7

The Lie Alcohol Told Me:
"Alcohol Washes Away the Pain"

The Truth I Figured Out:
I Can Deal with My Trauma with Clear Eyes and a Clear Head

Recently I read a story about Jesse Lingard, an English football player, who came up in the Premier League with Manchester United, arguably the most famous professional sports franchise in the world. Lingard joined United's acclaimed youth academy at the age of seven, the same age I was when I was eating cereal in front of the television set watching morning cartoons in my tighty-whities. He and I are not the same, obviously, but he and I do share a few things in common. Now, I don't know much about English football. To tell you the truth, reading the story was probably the first time I had even heard of Lingard. But I'll tell you what. I'm definitely going to remember his name and his incredible and inspiring courage in the face of circumstances that might have crushed anyone else.

Despite his longtime (and well-documented) success with United, appearing in more than two hundred matches, Lingard began to struggle with his game. It happens to every athlete: the ups and downs over the course of an otherwise respectable career. But Lingard couldn't get out of his slump. The English press savaged him, and the fans turned on him. He knew his time with United, the only club he ever knew, was coming to an unceremonious end, which caused him to doubt his talents more compulsively and, for the first time probably in his life, question his future in the game he loved. This isn't what grabbed my attention, though. What caught my attention was how Lingard's struggles on the pitch, as they call the field in football, followed him home. At night, alone and with circular thoughts and insecurities whirling around his head, Lingard started drinking to, in his words, "try and take the pain away." A guest on the popular English podcast *The Diary Of A CEO*, Lingard opened up about his struggles with drinking. "I needed something to try and take the pain away," he said. "And put me at ease somehow. I was drinking before bed, having a nightcap. I look back now and think, 'What was I doing that for?' I was trying to forget what was going on. But it makes it ten times worse."[1]

Exacerbating his problems, Lingard explained, was his mother's own mental health struggle. In 2019, as his play dropped off, his mother was admitted to a hospital for depression. While she was away, Lingard had to look after his two younger siblings. "The depression was so bad she couldn't really cope anymore, and she needed to go away and get help. But leaving me with my little sister who was eleven at the time, and my little brother who was fifteen, for me, I was still going through my own things as well. So, I wasn't really the big brother they wanted at the time. I just wasn't there mentally."

Although he's hardly a household name here in the United States, Lingard has a lot of what we used to call "down-home" wisdom, some lessons worth sharing around the kitchen table. In my experience, the need to drink to "wash away the pain" is a sure sign that you're addicted. But it's also a sign that you haven't adequately addressed a specific trauma. Instead, you're using alcohol as a coping mechanism. While Lingard was struggling in football, his mother was in the hospital, and he was in charge of his siblings, something he wasn't emotionally able to do. Turning to alcohol every night, he thought he had found a way to get through it. Thankfully, he recognized what he was trying to do.

I get it—drinking to forget your troubles makes a lot of sense. At least at first. This is basically what you and I have been told most of our lives. When we're faced with stressful situations, all of our problems seem to happen all at once. It suddenly seems like everything is an emergency, a deafening alarm in our heads. Why wouldn't we want to quiet that alarm? And why not turn to alcohol if it helps us turn down the volume or ignore this alarm completely? I mean, that's what we've always been told alcohol does. What we aren't told, however, is how turning to alcohol to wash away the pain is the express lane to addiction. Instead of practicing healthy habits, we're drinking to cope. Rather than trying to thrive, we're drinking to get by, which prevents us from recognizing that all of these stress-inducing moments we keep running into are really just symptoms of some deeper wound, some lingering trauma.

But don't think for a second that just because you had a great childhood or never experienced trauma in your life that you can't get addicted. Thirty percent of addicts say they had good childhoods. They are addicted to alcohol simply because it is a highly addictive substance: once you consume enough, anyone can and will get addicted.

I was part of the 70 percent that experienced trauma. But, up until recently, I had no clue I had an unconscious fear of abandonment until I removed the fog of alcohol from my mind. After I had been alcohol-free for a year, my ex-wife said she wanted to separate, which triggered my unconscious fear of abandonment and spiked my anxiety. For three days, I had an existential crisis, followed, eventually, by a spiritual awakening wrapped up in a big ball of wild psychosis. Everything came to a head at once, and it was far too much for me to handle. But, in the end, is there a difference between a breakdown and a breakthrough? Not in my experience. During my stay in a mental health treatment center, I tried to process the experience and figure out exactly what happened to me. I now believe my mind was, over the course of thirty days, shedding the previous thirty years of being numbed down by alcohol. It was an intense and incredible experience, one in which I was finally able to identify and start addressing the original trauma that I spent most of my life trying to wash away with alcohol: witnessing my father beat my mother as a five-year-old and being abandoned by him.

Basically, I lost my true self trying to self-medicate this childhood trauma that was buried deep in my memory, held there by my unconsciousness and my addiction to alcohol. As I grew older, I started to experience more of the long-term effects of this trauma. This made it harder to focus on the present, which only increased my need to keep drinking. Added to the normal stress of everyday life, I found myself drinking to excess more regularly, including daylong binges on the golf course followed by all-night dinner parties. Eventually, I came to recognize how limiting this approach is. It stopped me from dealing with issues and prevented me from experiencing the full spectrum of human emotions, leaving me even more vulnerable to alcohol's pernicious claims. But, like Lingard, I believed alcohol would quiet the alarm ringing in my head because that's the only thing we've ever been told. Drinking may have been the "solution" you turned to, but the truth is, it only makes things worse.

Rather than empowering us to address and heal our original traumas, drinking only exacerbates symptoms of trauma. It can contribute to posttraumatic symptoms and increase irritability, depression, and anxiety. Unaddressed trauma creeps into our sleep, and drinking disrupts it, a brutal combination that imprisons us in a vicious cycle of self-recrimination and self-sabotage. Our irritability increases, along with our impatience, anxiety, alienation, and dissatisfaction—all of which make us want to drink even more. The twin threats of unaddressed trauma and out-of-control drinking promote careless behavior and can cause new traumas.

Research on substance abuse finds a strong correlation between traumatic experiences and heavy-drinking behaviors. Surveys found that more than half of heavy drinkers have experienced childhood trauma.[2] This does not mean that trauma is necessary to create addiction; three out of ten heavy drinkers who didn't experience childhood trauma still abuse alcohol.[3] When someone finds temporary pain relief through alcohol, they will slowly increase their use of the substance until they can't go without it. Trauma or not, anyone can become dependent on an addictive substance. But if you've had childhood trauma in your life, you are more susceptible to getting addicted to alcohol in an attempt to deaden, numb, and kill the psychological pain.

YOUR FRONTAL LOBE, FOR STARTERS

You remember the old television ad with the fried egg: "This is your brain on drugs." I only wish it had said, "This is your brain on drugs, including alcohol."

If you want to know what is really happening to your brain when you try to drink away the pain, know this: when you consume alcohol, your frontal lobe becomes deadened and numb. This is what leads to "disinhibition," also known as poor decision-making. Your frontal lobe is responsible for weighing options, making decisions, performing evaluations, and expressing your personality. When you continuously deaden and numb this area of your brain, you're going to experience some flawed cognitive functioning. And, as we learned earlier, you're going to stop behaving like yourself. Again, alcohol doesn't make you fit in; it makes you forget who you are.

All alcohol does for the pain is add fuel (literal ethanol fuel) to the fire. Scientists now know the mechanism that explains why alcohol gives you both a high and a low. As we learned in the previous chapter, alcohol feels good because it releases GABA, which causes you to feel relaxed and calm. (Xanax does the same thing.) Alcohol also releases dopamine, the same way heroin does. It also pumps endorphins through your system, in much the same way cocaine does. The flood of these neurotransmitters creates a brief euphoric effect, but when you reach 0.05 percent blood alcohol content or higher, the negative effects start to take over. You feel depressed, exhausted, and uncomfortable. For the average person, this translates into two beers. Let me repeat that: two beers. The neurotransmitters that made you feel good start to run out and, if you want to restore your "normal" emotional functioning, you have to replenish them. Rebalancing your brain chemicals can take days, during which time you have to deal with increased anxiety and emotional pain.

According to John Mendelson, a clinical professor of medicine at the University of California in San Francisco, alcohol only helps you relax because it's kinking up our central nervous system. "Alcohol floods the brain with dopamine, creating feelings of euphoria. It also inhibits judgment and memory," he recently told Psych Central. "Together, these effects can temporarily relieve feelings like sadness and stress."[4]

Temporary, mind you—not permanent.

"You may experience momentary relief from emotional pain

when you drink alcohol. For a few minutes or hours, the burden of your grief could feel a bit lighter," Mendelson stressed. "But when the alcohol wears off, and the negative emotions come rushing back, you may feel even worse than you did before."

In other words, abusing alcohol as a coping mechanism only compounds the problem and sinks you deeper into the Alcohol Matrix. For most people in the Alcohol Matrix, drinking lets them temporarily quiet scary things like fear, shame, and vulnerability, all of which are symptoms of a deeper, underlying trauma. Those people are running away from their problems and their root causes, just as I was. Quieting those alarms sounding in our head sure does work in the moment, but eventually those alarms overwhelm us, as Jesse Lingard's story illustrates. Until we start to address the root causes of our addictions, we'll never start to get control of our emotions. We'll never be able to live freely and openly in the present moment.

The only way to get out of psychological pain or trauma is to be vulnerable and go through it without being under the influence of alcohol or drugs. You cannot go under (using a depressant like alcohol), over (using a stimulant like cocaine), or around (using a stimulant/depressant like cannabis) any psychological pain or trauma. You have to go through.

Speaking of cannabis, in the introduction I mentioned that the word *sober* means being subdued, somber, serious, solemn, grave, and restrained. Although I do have my ups and downs, I am very rarely doing any of those things, and I am definitely not restrained! At my truest essence I am joy, ease, and lightness. That's why I never say that I or anyone else is sober: I say alcohol-free.

I love to get out of my everyday consciousness with a daily meditation, and, on extremely rare occasions (about once every three years), get out of my everyday consciousness and partake in plant medicine. Therefore, technically, I am not sober in that way either. As Sting once said, "I don't think psychedelics are the answers to the world's problems, but they could be a start."

A serious disclaimer here: I do not condone or believe that any kind of recreational, "partying" use of psychedelics is healthy at all. It can be very dangerous. Make absolutely sure you consult with your doctor and that you are in a safe setting under the care of experienced, intentional professionals if you ever do any psychedelics.

Anyway, I have known since college that I am one of those people who, under the influence of cannabis in any form, curls up into a ball in the corner of the room, doesn't talk to anyone, and thinks over and over, *Why?*—an incessant torrent of meaningless, painful thought. Yet, about once every three years since college, someone has been able to talk me into trying cannabis with them in some different form. Each time their sales pitch has something to do with how it is a fun, different crystal, wax, tincture, hybrid, purple strain, or whatever. It sounds great each time, and I get peer pressured into trying it.

Ninety percent of the time it is not at all enjoyable for me, but six years ago, on Christmas Eve, my brother-in-law talked me into trying gummies. I told him that I only wanted a tiny bit, and he said his gummies were not strong at all, so I should take two for them to have any effect.

Fast-forward to an hour later, and I was stoned and reading *'Twas the Night Before Christmas* to my three- and four-year-old girls while all the other adults were downstairs. The three of us ended up having a one-hour, full-fledged, intense conversation about life. What came out of this conversation was that those little stinkers—I mean, angel girls—knew exactly what was going on, and I had been treating them like babies until this point. It took me getting out of my ordinary consciousness to see them, really be able to listen to them, and fully realize their new level of consciousness.

Now, mind you, "life" that night for the girls meant only one thing: Santa Claus. They asked me if I really believed in Santa, and I said, "Of course I believe in Santa! All I know is that I have always believed in everything about Santa, and every year I receive presents on Christmas. You know how Santa Claus is magic and only seems to have a human body but can slide down any chimney on Earth and not get hurt? Well, did you know that when one of you was only one year old and the other was in your mom's belly, we all got to go to the church in Italy where Saint Nicholas, Santa Claus, is said to be buried? He lives forever now by the power of our hearts and minds."

I am not a Bible thumper, but on this holiest of eves, the spirit of my Grandma Weezie, who taught children's Bible school for sixty-five years, came through me and said to the girls, "It is like Jesus, who was said to have been born on this night 2018 years ago. No one has ever found his bones, but we know for sure that he was walking on this earth with us for many years. He invited us to love God above all else and love one another as ourselves, then he suffered and died on the Cross for us. We now know that we do not need to suffer like he did, that we are forgiven when we really apologize for making a mistake, and that we are eternally and unconditionally loved by Him."

I can assure you that I would not have had that conversation with my girls while I was drunk on alcohol. As a matter of fact, I probably would not have read them a Christmas Eve bedtime story. I would have been downstairs with an extra-stiff eggnog bourbon in my hand, watching sports. For me, a touch of plant medicine (that is not rotten and toxic) on a rare occasion can be a good way to see things in a different light.

Even though cannabis is legal almost everywhere now, be sure you are careful with it. As with any drug, it can be highly addictive if you consistently reach out to it for comfort or use it in a compulsive way. Don't trade one addiction for another, and if you currently use cannabis *and* drink, it is time to cut both of them out and face yourself fully substance-free, once and for all.

Once your brain is not dead and numb from alcohol flowing through it on a consistent basis, it will gain most of its senses back. And it might press the fast-forward button, leaping your consciousness from one level to the next. This can be through a spiritual awakening, existential crisis, mental breakdown, or some combination of those. The three-day psychosis/spiritual awakening that I went through was one of the most incredible and painful experiences of my life, and I have gained so much from it. It just would have been nice if someone had warned me that might happen!

Well, I'm here to tell you to expect it, and that you're going to be okay.

People can and do change inside—*if* their consciousness is not numbed down by alcohol like mine was for thirty years. When psychological pain comes up, people do the natural thing, which is to reach for comfort. That comfort is often alcohol. It temporarily alleviates pain, yet it numbs your nervous system and all of your senses, both physical and mental.

But pain is at once the ultimate guide and primary warning signal that something is wrong. If we can't feel pain, we're not able to learn and grow. When your mind and all of your senses are numbed by alcohol, you cannot sense the pain, so your body and mind think everything is okay. Becoming alcohol-free has enabled me to really feel the psychological pain when it comes up. And I mean *really* feel it.

I have learned to lean into the pain instead of immediately

reaching for beer and wine. By no longer numbing out, I can finally see where the pain is coming from. I can begin to ask myself why I am having this anxiety, depression, insecurity, and/or fear, get vulnerable and ask for help from others, know the root cause, and work on it from there. Being alcohol-free has enabled me to take a deep, hard look in the mirror and begin to heal those unconscious wounds that I didn't know were still there. I feel so much more at peace now than I ever did while I was drinking. When it comes to emotional or mental pain/trauma (big or small), we must lean into the pain.

This, my friends, is the key to how we will truly stop all our suffering. By not covering up the psychological pain with a liquid drug, you will instead learn to lean into the bed of nails you are lying on. Once you have the courage to not reach for an external substance, you will be able to feel the pain and finally see why you are having it (usually from childhood trauma, but not always), and you can go into the pain and cure it once and for all.

If you experience a challenging mental or emotional shift after you stop drinking, know that you are not alone. The best thing is to get immediate professional help. In fact, it's even better if you start out with a therapist or doctor on your side who knows that you are becoming alcohol-free, or coaching groups like 100% U, which you can find at www.WeAretheAFR.org. Rather than drinking to wash away the pain, you can start to confront reality while mentally and physically readjusting to life without alcohol.

Now that I've said all that, you might be afraid of this possibility. That's okay. Staring down underlying trauma, depression, or anxiety while stone-cold conscious is hard and scary. But it's *not* a bad thing! Whether you cover them up or not, they're still there. And they're most likely at least part of why you started drinking in the first place. And, at this stage in your life, you realize trying to wash them away with alcohol hasn't done a damn thing to fix them. Getting these root issues out in the open empowers you to begin to heal those issues instead of slapping an addictive, toxic Band-Aid on them. You can see yourself in a real way, get real help, and finally begin working on those underlying struggles. As you start to rid your body and mind from poison, you can start to reckon with your personal history and core emotional traumas.

CHAPTER 8

The Lie Alcohol Told Me:
"One Drink Won't Kill You"

The Truth I Figured Out:
Not Drinking Improved My Physical, Mental, Spiritual, and Financial Well-Being

Recently, after not having a drop of alcohol in my mouth for two years, I went on a trip to Europe. I was with a friend who wanted to go on a wine tasting tour, and I do love a European winery (or any winery, for that matter). The views, grapevines, smells, food, and conversations are delightful. The exception is the addictive rotten-fruit liquid, more popularly known as wine.

On the tour, the sommelier kept taking sips of the wine and spitting it out. He explained to me in a heavy Italian accent that he no longer actually drank the wine because it "make a di' trouble at homa." But he loved his job and didn't want to lose it.

I told the sommelier, "*Anche io*. Me, too," sharing that I was just there with my friend who loved wine, and that I did not drink alcohol either, but I did drink nonalcoholic beers and wished there was a good nonalcoholic wine.

The kind sommelier suggested I should try wine like he did and spit it out after tasting it. I thought about that and agreed that just like using alcohol as an antiseptic on the skin, there should not be an issue with tasting the wine and then spitting it out, since the problems occur when the addictive toxin is consumed and absorbed into the bloodstream and the brain.

I was already having a great time on the tour, socializing with others from around the world, and I was very excited to join in on the tastings as well. In my addiction days, I had spent an unfortunate amount of time, money, and energy on guzzling, discussing, and researching wine. Being able to share my "expert" thoughts about the wine was going to make me feel even more a part of the group!

The sommelier poured a very expensive Chardonnay into the glass. The other eight people who were on the tasting tour had already tried it and praised it.

"Subtle hints of butter and crisp notes of pear."

"Smooth and oaky."

"Vanilla with English pudding."

I began the tasting process. I swirled the light-yellow liquid around in my glass and held the glass high in the air to see the viscosity. I then put the glass to my nose to take in as much of the smell as I could. Everything seemed normal and nice.

Until I tasted it.

Once the wine touched my tongue, my mind and mouth exploded with horror. I tried not to show how much I didn't like it. *It's like jet fuel!* my mind shouted while my tongue and mouth burned. I swished the wine around in my mouth to make sure my tasting technique was correct. But my senses were engulfed with fuel fumes, bad taste, and a burning sensation. My mind flashed red poison signs at me until I finally listened and spit the mouthful out.

I guess I was able to hide my discomfort because the sommelier asked me what I was tasing.

"Uhh . . . alcohol. What is the alcohol content of this

Chardonnay?" I asked.

He held up the bottle and said, "Dis' one, oh, t'is a light one, just a twelve percento." He was correct; wine's alcohol by volume (ABV) ranges from about 11 percent to 18 percent, so it was on the very low end. I asked my friend and the rest of the tasting group if they thought it tasted like it had a high alcohol content, and they all said no. But after two years of not having tasted alcohol, it was all I could taste in a high-end Chardonnay that everyone else enjoyed.

My trip to the vineyard reminded me of the many lessons I learned about alcohol once I started making my way out of the Alcohol Matrix. The most immediate lesson is that I don't like the taste of alcohol! I didn't like it when my grandfather let me sip his whiskey when I was six, and I don't like it now. It literally tastes like poison. And that's true about alcohol, no matter where you drink it or how it's packaged for market. It doesn't taste good, and it certainly isn't good for you. Neither an idyllic setting nor the most attractive label should distract from the fact that the prettily packaged poison you're drinking is rotting your bank account, your physical health, and your emotional and spiritual well-being.

I doubt this will come as any real surprise, but let me be clear: there is absolutely nothing healthy about alcohol. Nothing. No matter how many advertising and marketing campaigns try to sell you the nonsense that those new, popular hard seltzers contain "zero calories from sugar" or how many lifestyle publications proclaim clear liquor is "healthier" than dark liquor, alcohol is simply not healthy, at all.

Here's a little math for you. Don't worry, though, this one's easy. In fact, the answer is always the same, no matter how many times you crunch the numbers or try to fudge them. Remember in elementary school, probably when you were eight or nine years old, when your math teacher told you any number multiplied by zero always equals zero? I loved that lesson, probably because I always remembered the answer. My teacher, Ms. Baker, could have put the most convoluted equation on the blackboard and I would have aced it, as long as it included a zero. While my skinned-knee classmates sweated about order of operations—the dreaded PEMDAS—I confidently raised my hand and answered proudly, "The answer is zero, Ms. Baker."

Well, you can apply that same lesson to alcohol. Let's count how many positive effects alcohol has on your physical health.

The answer is zero.

Someone could ask how many positive effects a beer or glass of wine has on your physical health, or how many positive effects a screwdriver or Bloody Mary or vodka and soda have on your physical health. As long as the equation includes the word *alcohol,* the answer is always zero.

THERE'S NO SUCH THING AS A HEALTHY COCKTAIL

Of course, that doesn't stop bartenders and mixologists trying to trick (sorry, upsell) patrons with healthy-sounding drinks like pomegranate martinis or blueberry vodka. Again, there is nothing healthy about alcohol. Blending liquid poison with fresh organic fruit and jalapeno slices doesn't turn alcohol into a health elixir. A body-conscious drinker might justify ordering an açai highball because it's made with superfoods, so it *seems* like they're drinking a salad. Although açai berries do have incredible health benefits, those same incredible health benefits are cancelled out as soon as they're added to alcohol. Big Alcohol markets their seltzer products as low-calorie, all-natural serums that will get you drunk without the unwanted effects of beer, wine, and liquor. White Claw commercials call their cocktail "sparkling water with alcohol" as if it's clean, clear, and hydrating like a bottle of Perrier. Their marketing campaign aims to sell consumers on the idea that White Claw is healthy, but they over-look one crucial detail: sparkling water doesn't cause cancer or two hundred other diseases. Alcohol does. That beautiful bottle of bubbly water? It's poisoned with ethanol.

The scientific truth is that alcohol is ethanol, and ethanol is alcohol. A drink with 5 percent alcohol/ethanol is the same as any other drink with 5 percent alcohol/ethanol. The ingredi-ents of a specific alcohol-based drink—grapes, wheat, barley, agave, potatoes, rice, and hops—certainly contain different compounds, but the alcohol/ethanol derived from that rotten fruit or vegetable is the exact same addictive, cancer-causing substance. There is zero difference between the alcohol/ethanol of a light beer and that of a red or white wine, dark whiskey or rum, clear vodka or tequila, hard seltzer, or any other type of alcoholic drink.

When a label says ABV, that percentage is what you really need to know about the "health value" of that drink. Instead of ABV, I prefer to measure it by what I call addictive carcinogen by volume, or ACBV. Ambassadors for premium, expensive wines advertise their products as good for the heart and a great way to avoid the headaches of cheaper alcohols. However, "organic" wines are still more than 11 percent ACBV. A vintner based in the United Kingdom wants you to believe its toxic ethanol product is healthier than other ethanol products: "Despite the alcohol content, wine has long been associated with various ben-efits to your health when consumed in moderation. What a lot of people aren't aware of is the health benefits of organic wine when compared to conventional wine. . . . The key to avoiding harmful chemical content and healthier wine drinking lies in switching to organic wine. It comes as an excellent option for health-conscious wine drinkers who fear they are consuming harmful artificial additives when drinking conventional, super-market wines." Each of these sentences includes the word *health* or *healthier*! At least the rambling and erroneous sentence all begins with, "Despite the alcohol [poison] content . . ."[1]

Biodiesel might be better for the environment than petroleum-based fuel, but I think we can all agree that if you drank either, you would still end up in the ER. Apply this same reasoning to ethanol infused with organic fruits and vegetables: though it might taste better, it doesn't mean it's a liquid shot of great health. When you drink alcohol, you consume empty calories at the rate of at least a hundred calories per drink. There are a hundred calories in every shot, and the standard eight-ounce pour of light beer and five-ounce pour of red wine are both more than a hundred calories. Some sugary wines and craft beers can have over two hundred calories per eight-ounce serving. That's 10 percent of your recommended daily calorie intake in one glass. Those empty calories are broken down into simple sugars, which collect as fat and show up on your body in unflattering ways.

When I was drinking, my joints would hurt every time I worked out, especially my knees and shoulders. I accepted that I was getting old, and my joints would probably ache for life. Then I stopped drinking the poison that was dehydrating my body and inflaming my joints. The pain went away, my joints healed up between workouts, and I lost twenty pounds without changing anything except not consuming ethanol. I literally became lighter on my feet. Because I was putting less stress on my joints, they kept improving. I never felt this good with alcohol consistently running through my body. Alcohol is an anti-superfood. If you just cut this one thing, you'll have health benefits across the board. If your only diet is not drinking for a hundred days, you will most likely lose a significant amount of weight. Having lost

10 percent of my body weight just from becoming alcohol-free, I went from drinking-dad bod back to modeling bod.

Alcohol affects more than your body's weight or shape, unfortunately.

Alcohol is the number one killer for men ages nineteen to fifty-nine, according to the WHO.[2] Alcohol is responsible for three million deaths every year.[3] That's 5.3 percent of all deaths! To put that in perspective, when Covid was at its peak and we shut down the world, it killed 1.8 million people. If we want to save more people each year, all we must do is wear a mask when alcohol is around. And keep in mind that this figure only counts fatalities; it doesn't include those who lost their homes, families, jobs, or health because of alcohol consumption. Overall, according to the WHO, 5.1 percent of disease and injury around the world is attributable to alcohol.[4] In people aged twenty to thirty-nine years—men and women in the prime of life—approximately 13.5 percent of total deaths are attributable to alcohol.[5] There are also some stark gender differences in alcohol-related mortality and morbidity as well as alcohol consumption. Alcohol-attributable deaths among men amounts to about 8 percent of all global deaths, whereas it only amounts to less than 3 percent of all deaths among women. It's probably no coincidence that men drink more alcohol, per capita, than women around the world. According to the WHO, alcohol consumption among men in 2016 was an average of about 5 gallons, compared with an average of 1.8 gallons among women.[6]

WARNING: LABELS

Take a look at a bottle of alcohol. On it, you'll find a favorite disclaimer of mine near the end of the bottle's warning label. It says, "*may* cause health problems." *May? Might? Could? Really!* When has alcohol/ethanol *not* been toxic? When was alcohol/

ethanol *not* a carcinogen? It may not have been *listed* as a carcinogen before 1988, but it was always a carcinogen whether we knew it or not. Alcohol has officially been known to be a carcinogen for more than thirty years, yet fewer than 30 percent of people today know that it causes cancer. And the ones who do, unfortunately, don't believe alcohol is all that bad, unlike smoking tobacco.

But the fact is that alcohol is listed as a Group 1 carcinogen, just like tobacco.[7] A carcinogen causes cancer. That's cause and effect. When you make the choice to drink, you are choosing to put a cancer-causing substance in your body. But we don't want to believe that alcohol actually causes cancer (or two hundred other diseases) like smoking does because of our addiction, advertising lies, industry lobbyists, and our collective unconscious belief that alcohol is life's great elixir. We want to drink our addictive, cancer-causing beverage in peace.

"Many people are aware that tobacco causes lung cancer," explained George Laking, medical director of the Cancer Society at the launch of the society's campaign to raise awareness in New Zealand about the link between alcohol and cancer. "However, there is still a huge stigma around the link between alcohol and cancer." Alcohol causes seven types of cancer, according to Laking. "However, New Zealanders are typically unaware that alcohol (even small amounts) can increase the risk of developing at least seven cancers, including mouth, pharynx, larynx, [esophagus], breast, bowel and liver cancer. Due to its high energy content, alcohol can contribute to weight gain and indirectly increase the risk of weight-related cancers."[8]

Put another way, he said, "There is really no safe level of alcohol consumption in relation to cancer."

Similarly, Susan Brink writes for NPR: "At least 4% of the world's newly diagnosed cases of esophageal, mouth, larynx, colon, rectum, liver and breast cancers in 2020, or 741,300 people, can be attributed to drinking alcohol, according to a study in the July 13 edition of *Lancet Oncology*." She goes on to explain how ethanol "breaks down to form a known carcinogen called acetaldehyde, which damages DNA and interferes with cells' ability to repair the damage."[9] An increase in hormone levels, including estrogen, is also caused by drinking alcohol. Cells get their signals from hormones to grow and divide. When cells divide more, there are a lot more chances for cancers to develop.

Not long after my dad's death from alcohol-induced cancer, one of my uncles told me that he had prostate cancer. We were at a winery together after my nephew's baptism. The priest who performed the baptism, and whom I admire and respect immensely, was drinking white wine with my uncle. The priest was fully aware that my uncle had prostate cancer and was about to begin radiation treatment. Watching my uncle drink that yellow-tinted ethanol, I was in complete horror. All I could see were cancer cells enjoying a liquid-poison swim party inside my uncle's prostate. Although I can't remember my words exactly, I definitely recall saying something to my uncle and the family priest about alcohol causing cancer. The priest took a large sip and said something about canon law. My whole body trembled with shock. I was so upset; I couldn't say anything else.

The next day I called my uncle. "Uncle, with all due respect, alcohol is ethanol. Alcohol has been one hundred percent proven to cause cancer. Alcohol is a level one carcinogen, which is the same level as cigarettes. *Please*, at a very minimum, do not drink any alcohol while you are going through your cancer treatment. I am sending you a bunch of nonalcoholic IPAs. When you feel like a cold beer, go for it. I have already lost a dad to cancer caused by alcohol. I am not losing an uncle to it as well."

Some people who drink alcohol just love to remind you that Jesus drank wine. They talk a lot about the Gospel story of Jesus turning water into wine at a wedding in Canaan. This is probably what the priest was thinking when he dismissed me. But do you think that after seeing all the science about alcohol/ethanol he would say that the wine of today is fine to drink on a regular, moderate, and responsible basis? Did Jesus ever mean for us to guzzle alcohol like we do today? I don't think so.

Beyond its link to cancer, alcohol can dramatically impact the health of your brain. Chronic drinking leads to a lack of thiamine (vitamin B1) in the brain. Thiamine is responsible for breaking down sugars and providing energy to the brain. Without it, you can develop Korsakoff syndrome, an irreversible condition marked by dying brain cells, slower levels of cognition, and large holes in your brain. Vital neurological areas, deprived of energy, begin to shrink. You will lose the ability to think, feel, and balance. Drinking thins out the corpus callosum, the bundle of nerves that connect the right and left hemispheres of the brain, which makes it difficult to pick up on social cues, including the recognition of facial expressions. Further, drinking alcohol can cause hippocampal atrophy, which leads to the inability to recall long-term memories. Let me repeat that: alcohol affects your ability to recall memories, even if you've only been drinking for a few years!

Here's the thing about researching alcohol: it's impossible not to come across new studies and statistics that don't run counter to everything we've ever been told about alcohol, from Madison Avenue to the federal government. A team from the University of Pennsylvania, for instance, recently analyzed data from more than 36,000 adults and found that light-to-moderate alcohol consumption was associated with reductions in overall brain volume.[10] As if that wasn't worrisome enough, the researchers found that the link between alcohol consumption and poor brain health grew stronger as the level of alcohol consumption grew. If, for instance, an average fifty-year-old increased his drinking from one alcohol unit (about half a beer) a day to two units (a pint of beer or a glass of wine), the associated change in the brain is the equivalent to aging two years.[11] Going from two to three alcohol units at the same age was like aging three-and-a-half years. "These findings contrast with scientific and governmental guidelines on safe drinking limits," said study coauthor Henry Kranzler, director of the Penn Center for Studies of Addiction. "For example, although the National Institute on Alcohol and Alcoholism recommends that women consume an average of no more than one drink per day, recommended limits for men are twice that, an amount that exceeds the consumption level associated in the study with decreased brain volume."[12]

LET'S TALK ABOUT YOUR LIVER

With the exception of the brain, the liver is the most complex organ in the body. Its functions include filtering toxins from the blood, aiding digestion of food, regulating blood sugar and cholesterol levels, and helping fight infection and disease.[13] A resilient organ, the liver can regenerate. Years of prolonged drinking, however, diminishes this ability, which can result in serious and permanent damage to the liver, including fatty liver disease, alcoholic hepatitis, and cirrhosis. Drinking to excess, even for just a few days, can lead to a buildup of fat in the liver. Drinking over a longer sustained period of time can lead to alcoholic hepatitis, a potentially serious condition unrelated to infectious hepatitis. According to the Mayo Clinic, most people who develop alcoholic hepatitis consumed more than seven glasses of wine, seven beers, or seven shots of spirits every day for at least twenty years.[14] Cirrhosis is when the liver becomes significantly scarred following years of alcohol abuse. A person who has alcohol-related cirrhosis and doesn't stop drinking has a less than 50 percent chance of survival beyond five years.[15] A 2021 study showed that among the 159,973 alcohol-associated liver disease hospitalizations in the United States, 83.7 percent had a primary diagnosis of alcohol-associated cirrhosis and 18.4 percent had a primary diagnosis of alcoholic hepatitis, with significantly higher hospitalization rates in men than women for both conditions.

You think bloodshot eyes after a night of drinking are bad? Far worse, and far creepier, are yellow eyes. As the liver becomes more damaged from ethanol, people lose the ability to clear out dead red blood cells that collect in the eyes and tinge them a lovely shade of yellow. Remember the bully in the movie *A Christmas Story*? "There he stood . . . Scut Farkus, staring out at us with his yellow eyes. He had yellow eyes! So help me God, yellow eyes!" Don't be a Scut Farkus.

With all these statistics, it's no wonder the WHO considers alcohol, which has at least a causal factor in more than two hundred disease and injury conditions, to be one of the most harmful substances on Earth, more dangerous than crack, heroin, and prescription painkillers.[16]

And this is to say nothing about alcohol's causal relationship with a range of mental and behavioral disorders and other noncommunicable conditions and injuries.[17]

Beyond health consequences, abusing alcohol carries significant social and economic losses. The total economic cost of alcohol abuse has been estimated to be $249 billion, according to the CDC.[18] The CDC projects that the economic impact to society is about $807 per person, per year.[19] Alcohol use disorder also effects employment, an essential part of the economy. Alcohol use disorder leads to disruptions caused by tardiness, absenteeism, worker turnover, and workplace conflict. It also causes a reduction in potential employees, customers, and taxpayer bases. That said, because the researchers acknowledged information on alcohol is often underreported or unavailable, and the study did not include other costs (such as pain and suffering due to alcohol-related injuries and diseases), the scope of this problem is likely larger.

What we can note, however, is that the unemployed drink alcohol at a significantly higher frequency than the employed and consume slightly higher amounts.[20] Unemployed people also had significantly higher rates of problematic or, in the words of one study, "high-dose" drinking patterns.[21]

Alcohol abuse is often a cause of homelessness. Nearly 70 percent of homeless people report that alcohol and/or drugs were a major reason for their becoming homeless.[22] This is a huge problem, and I firmly believe that if we ban alcohol advertising, we will help reduce homelessness dramatically. Although obtaining an accurate count is difficult, the Substance Abuse and Mental Health Services Administration estimates that in 2009, 38 percent of homeless people were dependent on alcohol and 26 percent abused other drugs. Substance abuse is much more common among homeless people than in the general population.[23] A 2008 survey by the United States Conference of Mayors asked twenty-five cities for their top three causes of homelessness. Substance abuse was the single largest cause of homelessness for single adults (reported by 68 percent of cities). Substance abuse was also mentioned by 12 percent of cities as one of the top three causes of homelessness for families.[24]

It's clear alcohol abuse can erode the health and well-being of the culture at large. Until we accept the scientific facts about alcohol/ethanol and ask ourselves, "Does alcohol benefit us?" we will never see honest warning labels on bottles and cans.

Instead, we will continue to suffer and watch our children and their children suffer and die in countless ways from drinking an addictive, health-destroying poison.

In the meantime, you don't need a degree in advanced mathematics to know that drinking alcohol is a lot more expensive than not drinking, especially in a world of hipster hangouts and hand-crafted drinks. Add sales tax and a tip to your tab and one drink can round out to a horrendous twenty dollars! And we all know we aren't just having one drink a night. The yearly cost of buying alcohol for a heavy drinker has been estimated to be up to $17,000. That might seem high, but my personal cost was about $12,000 a year. And—oh, yeah—the cost of one DUI can be up to $17,000! Not to mention the cost to your own mental health and medical bills. It might be difficult to quantify how expensive your own light, moderate, or heavy alcohol addiction can be, but it is never cheap, whether you're out tipping bartenders or at home tipping up that jug of bottom-shelf whiskey.

I have an alcohol-free app that currently says that I have been alcohol-free for three years and eight months, I have saved $40,860, money that I now spend guilt-free on retreats in exotic locations around the world with activities like surfing, golf, hiking, farm-to-table organic meals, yoga, meditation, massage, and many other incredible and healthy things.

The most awesome statistic the app shows, however, is its "time" tab. I used to spend an average of two hours per day either drinking or being under the influence of alcohol. In the past three years and eight months I have saved 2,724 hours, the equivalent of three months and twenty days of my life being more present and real with my young children—actually playing with them instead of pushing them off because I didn't feel like playing, either because I was too busy drinking or too hungover to engage. By the time my girls are both eighteen, I will have saved two full years of being present with them instead of being under the addictive influence of a poison. Two full years of their young lives!

If you are a parent, or want to be a parent, and that statistic doesn't jolt you into doing everything you can to overcome your alcohol addiction, then I don't know what will. It is by far the best part of living alcohol-free for me. And now that I have stopped consuming a cancer-causing poison, I have also dramatically increased my chances of living longer. Which means I will get to spend even more time with my girls when they're adult women—and, hopefully, with my future grandchildren.

I encourage you to pick up your phone right now, search in apps for "alcohol addiction recovery," and download an app. Enter details about your lifestyle to get a better picture of your time and money spent on alcohol. The process is simple, and the results are immediate. Type in something like, *I spend $13 a day buying two beers with tip and tax at the bar,* then sit back and watch your bank account grow every day for a year until you reach $4,745—nearly $5,000—in annual savings!

Alcohol costs you a ridiculous amount of time and money. Going alcohol-free will save your life, your relationship with your family, and a ton of money.

When you go alcohol-free, your heart, brain, liver, stomach, and skin will rejuvenate and function at optimal levels, boosting your mood and energy. The pounds will fall off your body as you reduce your calorie intake without even trying. You'll look good and feel great. You'll have more restful sleep and wake up with the energy of someone half your age who drinks.

I once spent the afternoon with the rock band Def Leppard. The singer, Joe Elliot, struck up a conversation with me. He told me about the time the band played in China and was supposed to be onstage at 7 p.m. sharp. Every fifteen minutes after 7, officials from the Chinese government kept coming to their hotel rooms and yelling at them to go perform. Joe told them, "We are an English rock band! We don't go onstage on time. We go when we f'ing feel like it."

As he put his cigarette out after telling me that story, he looked me up and down and asked me how he could get in shape.

"Maybe not be the lead singer of an English rock band," I said.

He laughed and nodded, then walked away.

The best response for anyone who asks why you don't drink is, "I feel a lot better when I don't drink." This disarms everyone. The reason they are drinking is to make themselves feel better, but deep down they know they are drinking poison and masking their psychological pain. When you say the exact opposite of what their unconscious mind believes, and you say the simple truth in a present, conscious way, there is nothing they can come back with that makes any sense.

DETOX TIMELINE: SIX MONTHS ALCOHOL-FREE

If you're paying attention to my own Detox Timeline, you'll probably guess that I hit the six-month mark on March 19, 2020, right around the start of the Covid-19 pandemic.

My ex-wife and I were in Angel Fire, New Mexico, with our daughters for spring break. When the schools started shutting down—along with pretty much everything else—we decided to stay there. I started homeschooling the kids while she worked from dawn to midnight, which I now believe was to avoid me. Even though I was feeling better physically, I was still blaming, shaming, and attacking her psychologically because I hadn't started the psychological work I needed to do to address my underlying traumas.

Oh, and we were also remodeling the house, which only added to the chaos. Life was suspended, and we were living in a half-finished home.

I never wanted a drink through any of it. I just kept up with my apps, meditations, and exercise. I leaned on my community and listened to Annie Grace's *This Naked Mind Podcast*.

I also practiced a lot of affirmations, which made me feel like I was in the *Saturday Night Live* skit "Daily Affirmations with Stuart Smalley." Stuart's famous line in his mock self-help show while looking in the mirror in his lavender button-down cardigan was, "I'm good enough, I'm smart enough, and doggone it, people like me."

Affirmations may sound woo-woo, but they have been scientifically proven to work wonders on reprogramming our minds. Psychologist Catherine Moore writes, "Positive affirmations require regular practice if you want to make lasting, long-term changes to the ways that you think and feel. The good news is that the practice and popularity of positive affirmations are based on widely accepted and well-established psychological theory." [25] I downloaded a consciousness-raising app called Motivation: Daily Quotes. You can choose all kinds of different categories like New Beginnings, Overthinking, Inner Peace, and so on, and set the app to send you an affirmation as many times a day as you wish.

Since the mind causes anxiety and depression, it can alleviate them as well. I do understand that for those with clinical depression, it is not as simple as choosing to be peaceful. I admire your courage and have so much compassion for you. Always remember that you are so much more than any diagnosis.

Although I can absolutely say I was feeling super clean—mentally, spiritually, and physically—six months in, I also want to admit that I was feeling *all* of my feelings, at every moment. The lows were pretty low, which I took as a great sign. It was probably one of the few times in my adult life when I wasn't hiding from tough feelings or hard truths by drinking myself numb.

Six months is when a lot of healing starts. It's painful, and a reminder of why you probably started drinking in the first place. Remember, though, to lean into the pain, instead of immediately reaching for beer and wine.

This is a big transition period. In addition to dealing with pain you likely haven't addressed, you'll also watch as your social circle changes. Old drinking buddies no longer want to hang out with you because you're alcohol-free, and you're trying to make new friends. You're creating a new life for yourself, finding new hobbies and new ways to fill your day.

Remember, this is what progress is like, even if it can feel a little scary.

PART IV

LIFE, LOVE, AND HAVING A BLAST, ALCOHOL-FREE

CHAPTER 9

The Lie Alcohol Told Me:
"You're the Problem, Not Alcohol"

The Truth I Figured Out:
I Am Not Defective or Incurable

I attended an AA meeting when I was ten years old. The room was so full of Big Tobacco cigarette smoke that I couldn't see clearly through the haze. My sinuses and throat burned. But I was there with my grandpa, whom I considered the coolest guy in the world. I always wanted to spend time with him—everyone around town did. He liked to hunt and fish, every country boy's dream. I can't count how many times I used to hop in his big ol' truck with him. Toss a line in Cedar Lake to catch some bass? *Abso-freakin'-lutely*. Run to the grocery store for Grandma? *Sounds fun*. Hand out tokens at the local AA meeting? *Sign me up*.

Grandpa was a happy, healthy, fun, social guy. I didn't know that he had stopped drinking around the time I was born. Sitting in the middle of his local AA group, hardly hip-high to the adults around me, I couldn't see anything but the life-loving, good-time-having, outdoors-enjoying man I idolized. He was perfect, exactly as he was. He was everything I wanted to be. What was he doing surrounding himself with a bunch of people who were addicted to alcohol?

When I got older, I learned he wasn't always like this. I started to hear more tales about his drinking days and addiction to alcohol from my relatives, each one a horror story. My grandpa's neighbors used to say he was the most miserable man in Canadian County. Without question, the most famous story was the one about the buried moonshine. People throughout the county were still talking about it when I was in high school! When my grandpa worked the fields at the ripe old age of fourteen, he would drink all day from a buried jar of moonshine. Back then he was behind a team of mules to till the soil, plant seeds, or harvest crops. He secretly kept a bottle buried in a certain patch of earth that he would pass on every lap. Whenever he reached his trove, he'd unearth the jar and take a drink. This was no sip of beer. This was backwoods, slap-yo'-momma, hyperpotent, blindness-inducing moonshine. By the end of the day, after working sunup to sundown, he was in an atrocious state. He'd lash out and get violent, but very few people knew why. He was good at covering his tracks.

My grandpa's abusive alcohol stories didn't make any sense to me. Here he was showing up to meetings, supporting and sponsoring others, and handing out thirty-day chips. How could such a kind, fun-loving, and generally nice guy turn into a monster after drinking alcohol? I had never seen that side of him. Grandpa didn't share his drinking experiences at the AA meetings when I was there. I suppose he had already shared his story with the group, and all these years later, he no longer had any interest in talking about his past. I also think he wanted me to see him for who he was after his addiction, not who or what he used to be.

When polite company talks about alcohol addiction, they often throw around terms like *incurable* or *diseased* or even *defective.* Grandpa wasn't any of those things, as far as I'm concerned. He certainly wasn't defective. Hell, the man I knew wasn't even defined by his addiction. I had no way of articulating this when I was ten, but I've since learned that anyone who has ever been addicted to alcohol (or any other substance) is so much more than their addiction.

Although there's no right or wrong away to kick an addiction, I do think my biggest issue with most traditional recovery programs, including Alcoholic Anonymous, is how they preach to their members, explicitly or implicitly, messages that inadvertently stigmatize people with addictions and, in so doing, interfere (ironically) with their recovery. Members of AA, for instance, believe they will always be alcoholics, no matter how many years they go without drinking. I believed this until I read *This Naked Mind*, had my awakening from the Alcohol Matrix, and was completely cured (yes, cured) of my addiction to alcohol. Thanks to this experience, I learned that alcohol has always been an addictive substance. Getting hooked on an addictive substance is not a disease, and it's certainly not an incurable disease. The basic philosophy of AA is based on what I view as the false premise that addiction is a permanent state and, just as concerning, is solely the fault of an individual, a sign of inherent weakness. I call this false premise the defective theory, and as I've come to understand, any approach rooted in this theory leaves a lot to be desired.

Right before I sat down to write this chapter, a friend sent me a clip of *The Drew Barrymore Show.* I love Drew as much as anyone, but I have to admit, her talk show doesn't feature heavily in my viewing rotation. My friend, though, suspected that Drew's interview with actor Jason Ritter, John Ritter's son, would resonate with me. It did. Jason was on the show with his wife, New Zealand actress Melanie Lynskey, the star of *Yellow-jackets*. Drew asked an anodyne question about how they met, standard fare for talk shows these days. I was just about to close the tab, because I really have no interest in celebrities' meet-cute stories. What caught my attention was Jason's demeanor. Before he spoke, I could already tell he was nervous.

"I knew how incredible Melanie was early on," he said. "But it's not as cute a story as you would like to think."

He continued, and I started to realize he wasn't nervous. He was embarrassed. I knew exactly where this was going.

"It was messy and interesting and weird. But mixed in . . . [I] was dealing with some alcoholism issues. And so, yeah, there was a lot . . . I knew how amazing she was, and I thought she would be incredible for someone who deserved her, basically, and I didn't feel like I was that person. . . . It was only after like maybe a year [of] not drinking when I started to go, 'Oh, maybe I can promise some things to someone else. Maybe I can be this person.' It's been like a slow burn. I knew that she was incredible. It was working on myself enough to feel like maybe I could be the one for her, too."

I stand and applaud Jason's vulnerability. I know how hard it is to admit that you're addicted to alcohol. And I only had to admit that to my friends and family. Jason was owning his addiction on national television. At the same time, I felt for him, too. As I watched him tell his story, I could see that he was still carrying the heavy weight of unnecessary shame that too often comes with beating addiction.

This is a great illustration of what I mean by the defective theory. Yes, it's absolutely necessary to own your own behavior and start reckoning with your addiction. But you should never be ashamed about your addiction, because it isn't your fault. Nor should you feel as if you're somehow defective, or inherently less than, for getting addicted. From the moment we're born to the moment we realize we're addicted to alcohol, we're encouraged to drink. In my view, at a certain point, anyone who regularly drinks will get addicted to alcohol. It's a matter of when, not who. Just because you're addicted to alcohol doesn't mean you're defective or incurable or unworthy or unlovable. It just means you're human.

I wish AA and other recovery groups focused on this. Look, AA helped so many people in my life, from my grandpa and dad to my brother, Darron. The list of Dunbars who owe their recovery to AA is probably as long as the merch line at Coachella. My concern, though, is that the AA model and other similar models of recovery are outdated and not as effective as they could be.

THE HISTORY OF AA

I want to share a little bit about AA and its founding. Bill Wilson and Dr. Robert Holbrook Smith, also known as Dr. Bob. Wilson and Dr. Bob started AA in 1935. The exact date was June 10, 1935, the same day Dr. Bob had his last beer.[1] For most of their lives, both Wilson and Dr. Bob struggled with their alcohol addiction. No matter how many times they tried to give it up, or no matter how long they went without drinking, they continued to relapse. When they met, Wilson was traveling through Akron, Ohio, where Dr. Bob was living at the time. Fearing another relapse, Wilson inquired about local "alcoholics" who might help him fight his temptation. That's how he met Dr. Bob. Dr. Bob helped Wilson stay sober and invited him to stay with him in Akron. A month later, Dr. Bob relapsed, and Wilson helped him get sober, though not before he gave him a few drinks to ward off the shakes. The next morning, June 10, Wilson had a beer to calm his nerves before performing an operation at the local hospital. Together, they worked to come up with a system of recovery. The problem of addiction, as they understood it, was that there are people who seem to be able to handle their drinking, and there are people who seem to not be able to handle their drinking.

Informing their approach was the work of Dr. William Duncan Silkworth. As director of the Charles B. Towns Hospital for Drug and Alcohol Addictions, Dr. Silkworth recognized that addiction is a result of moral turpitude or a weak constitution. He believed, given the evidence in front of him, that addiction was pathological, specifically a hypothetical allergy. "It is our purpose to show that there is a type of alcoholism characterized by a definite symptomatology and a fixed diagnosis indicative of a constant and specific pathology; in short, that true alcoholism is a manifestation of allergy," Dr. Silkworth wrote in his famous paper, "Alcoholism as a Manifestation of an Allergy."[2] In this same paper, Dr. Silkworth also writes: "The majority of people who drink alcohol apparently do with impunity."

In *This Naked Mind*, Annie Grace shares an excerpt from a letter that Dr. Silkworth wrote to Bill Wilson: "We believe . . . that the action of alcohol on these chronic alcoholics is a manifestation of an allergy; that the phenomenon of craving is limited to this class [of people] and never occurs in the average temperate drinkers. These allergic types can never safely use alcohol in any form at all; and once having formed the habit [they have] found they cannot break it, once having lost their self."

Meanwhile, modern psychology, still very much in the Dark Ages in the 1930s, had barely touched on the idea of the collective unconscious. Medical doctors were still performing lobotomies—they thought it was a good idea to just chop out part of someone's brain if they had a mental illness. The prevailing belief was that a mental illness meant there was something out of whack in the brain, a faulty part in there that needed to be replaced or removed. Another fun psychiatric procedure that was common in early psychiatry was electroconvulsive therapy, commonly known as shock therapy. Shock therapy was the universal treatment for mental illnesses back then, but when new technologies like CT scans and MRIs emerged in the 1970s, such methods were highly criticized for their poor efficacy at treating mental illness.

Look, I'm not trying discredit anyone, especially a doctor. I'm not an MD; but I do think it's entirely fair to point out that doctors in the 1930s, no matter how radical a particular theory might have been, were simply working with the best information and technology available to them at the time. They simply didn't have sufficient evidence to refine their theories about mental and physical ailments and illnesses.

Dr. Silkworth had to come up with a best guess as to why some people seemed to be able to handle their drinking and some people seemed to not be able to do so. What he came up with—and what Wilson and Dr. Bob later codified as part of their AA program—is what I call the defective theory of alcohol. In his famous paper "Alcoholism as a Manifestation of an Allergy," Dr. Silkworth also wrote the following: "The majority of people who drink alcohol apparently do so with impunity . . . . Such people drink from choice and not from necessity. They find in alcohol a pleasant stimulation, a relief from anxieties, an increased warmth of conviviality. It is not a dominant factor in their lives. They are normal people, mentally and physically, to all intents and purposes."[3]

In The Big Book, AA's bible, is the following passage: "Rarely have we seen a person fail who has thoroughly followed our path. Those who do not recover are people who cannot or will not give themselves to this simple program, usually men and women who are constitutionally incapable of being honest with themselves.

There are such unfortunates. They are not at fault; they seem to have been born that way."[4]

Dr. Silkworth pointed the blame on "such unfortunates" rather than ever considering the actual source of the problem: alcohol. Why? Because, like everyone else, Dr. Silkworth, Dr. Bob, and Bill Wilson all believed that alcohol was addictive to only a defective few, like my grandpa, who succumbed to alcohol because of a hypothetical allergy.

It's my belief that alcohol is addictive to everyone. It's only a matter of when a person gets addicted. It's never a question of who gets addicted.

I also believe that any and all addicts are curable and do not need to treat their addiction as a chronic disease. Along with the defective theory, I question the idea that addiction is incurable, or that it needs to be a chronic problem for the rest of a person's life. The "alcoholic" believes that once they finally accomplish the feat of becoming alcohol-free, they have to manage their addiction every day, for the rest of their lives, one day at a time. It doesn't have to be that way. The hopeless belief that alcohol addiction is an incurable personality trait is a result of programming, not biological fact, and it sends the wrong message to addicts and social drinkers alike. Under this model, alcohol will still tempt and haunt you long after you've had your last drink, right up until your death. This causes people to resist and fear alcohol, which in turn gives alcohol *more* power. To paraphrase Eckhart Tolle: whatever you resist, persists.

CONSIDER THE SUCCESS RATE OF AA

Although the exact percentage is still up for debate, Cochrane Reviews, the gold standard for analyzing health research and what insurance companies rely on most, found that AA has a success rate of 42 percent.[5] Other studies suggest lower rates—sometimes as low as 5 percent—but I want to give AA the most credit possible. A success rate of 42 percent is great, if you're playing baseball. Hit .420, and you're headed to Cooperstown. But addiction isn't baseball. Failing nearly 60 percent of the time isn't a good success rate. Nor should it be acceptable. Keep in mind that those successful 42 percent are people who were at the absolute end of their rope, at rock bottom, and would do anything to get out of the pain and trauma of alcohol addiction. They finally and desperately turned themselves in at AA and proclaimed that they were "alcoholics" after everyone else had told them, and they came to believe that they were defective. Losing almost 60 percent of these people is not a good success rate at all. We can and will do better with the understanding that alcohol is addictive to everyone and that all addictions are curable.

ROCK BOTTOM

Another issue I have with AA is that it unintentionally encourages people addicted to alcohol to drink until they hit rock bottom, when they are finally able to accept that they're helpless in the face of this incurable disease. But, as Darron likes to remind me, "You don't have to ride the garbage truck all the way to the dump." Meaning, of course, that you don't have to wait until you have completely screwed up your life to quit. Darron rode the truck to the dump, got out, rolled around awhile, made friends with the rats, and stiffed the driver. "When I do something," he said, "I do it into the ground. When people tell me my art or my jokes or my different fandoms are 'too much,' I tell them, 'I know the word "too" and I know the word "much," but when you put them together like that, I have no idea what you're saying.'" Trying to stop drinking, Darron was admitted into a medically supervised detox eight times, and on two separate occasions he stayed in a thirty-day rehab facility. He also got two DUIs, including the one in his driveway, and stayed in a sober-living house for two-and-a-half years. He finally stopped drinking on March 12, 2004, thanks to AA, which worked for him: he was one of the fortunate 40 percent, along with my grandpa and my dad. A core belief of AA is that it supports any kind of treatment that can get and keep people alcohol-free. I share this belief. Even if it took so long for my brother to get there.

About a year and a half into being alcohol-free, I was talked into going to an AA meeting. Because of Covid, the meeting was held online. I logged on to experience firsthand what AA was all about for people addicted to alcohol, as opposed to just attending it as a kid with my grandfather. The kind and compassionate people in the meeting kept trying to get me to say, "Hi, my name is Dustin Dunbar, and I am an alcoholic." They tried about four times, but I just sat there, looking into the camera with a silent stare. The whole time I wanted to scream, "I am not an alcoholic! I used to be addicted to alcohol, but I'm not now!" Just like someone who used to be addicted to cigarettes and now *knows* they are disgusting, addictive, and deadly, I used to be addicted to alcohol and now *know* it is disgusting, addictive, and deadly. If a person does not have any desire whatsoever to drink alcohol, then that person is cured. They are not perpetually a "recovering alcoholic," as the defective theory maintains. They are someone who was once addicted to alcohol. Just like someone who was once addicted to cigarettes is no longer a "smokeaholic," *I am not an alcoholic!* I could drink alcohol just like any other person who is high functioning and drinks alcohol on a consistent basis, and I could drink it anytime I want to. I *choose* not to, because it is disgusting to me in the same way inhaling a cigarette is disgusting to me.

But just don't take my word for it. A study published in

Neuropsychopharmacology found evidence for compulsive alcohol-seeking behavior in rats.[6] But only *after* they've been forced to consume enough alcohol that they become addicted. A nonaddicted rat will never drink alcohol voluntarily. Think about that: rats will eat and drink literally everything, including feces, while happily swimming around in raw sewage, but they won't touch alcohol. The Okie farm boy in me just has to say it: rats will literally eat shit, but they won't drink alcohol! And this Okie farm boy knows a lot about rats. I had to conduct research on a ton of rats in grad school because they are so genetically similar to humans.[7]

Another telling and troubling fact is that all of the rats began to drink alcohol voluntarily after they had been force-fed enough of it to develop a physical addiction. After enough exposure, the addictive nature of alcohol turns healthy rats, who are instinctively smart enough to avoid alcohol, into addicts.[8] Or what AA insists on calling alcoholics.

The term *alcoholic* connotes that there is something permanently wrong with people who are addicted to alcohol. We have to realize that the term *alcoholic* is outdated and reinforces the idea that even if you're alcohol-free, alcohol still has power over you. When you call yourself and others who have overcome their alcohol addiction "alcohol-free," on the other hand, you are empowering yourself and empowering others. You're opting out of calling yourself and others "incurable, diseased alcoholics," and you acknowledge that past addicts don't drink alcohol because they simply don't want to drink an addictive carcinogen, not because they are broken or defective.

Saying you're alcohol-free creates an entirely different narrative. It makes it easier to talk about your past addictions without reliving the pain and guilt. You're not an alcoholic. You've wised up to the reality of what drinking does to your body and have removed the compulsive habit from your life. Living alcohol-free rather than as a recovering alcoholic is a recognition that you've evolved beyond alcohol and found greater peace and fulfillment when it is not in your life.

While doing research for this book, I did a couple of podcasts and interviewed many people who had overcome alcohol addiction. Some veterans of AA told me they thought my book would be a death sentence for some people in AA. They said I needed to be very careful with what I say because if people start to know that alcohol is truly a substance that anyone can get addicted to, they might not go to AA meetings anymore and it might kill them. But the idea that you need to continue to attend meetings for the rest of your life, even after you have zero cravings or desire to drink, is based on the defective theory.

I know AA helps some people, but it doesn't tell others the scientific truth about alcohol, and it doesn't truly cure their members. The false message that only a certain type of person can get addicted is literally killing people. Remove the defective theory and incurably diseased label, and AA can easily achieve both cures for their members and actual prevention of alcohol addiction. Here's what today's science concludes: Alcohol addiction does not occur from human defects, personality disorders, or some hypothetical addiction allergy. Alcohol is an addictive substance that anybody can and will get addicted to once they consume enough of it.

Some AA members said that my refutation of the defective theory could ruin AA. One literally told me not to tell the scientific truth. *Hurt me with the truth, but never comfort me with a lie.* This is what my girls and I say to one another when the truth is hard to hear, but we know in the end it is the right thing to say. AA will thrive and be far more successful at actually healing people if it evolves out of the defective theory.

In 1632, Galileo published a book about heliocentricity, the belief that the universe revolves around the sun. This was contrary to the prevailing belief within the Catholic Church that the universe revolves around Earth. Angered by Galileo's publication, the legal body of the Church summoned him to a trial. When Galileo asked the high priests to look through the telescope, they refused to look. Entertaining an alternate theory was not an option. The Church ruled that Galileo was committing heresy and jailed him for the rest of his life. In 1992, the Church finally recognized their wrong and officially apologized for their refusal to accept Galileo's scientific truth. It took more than three hundred years for the Church to admit that Galileo was right and to clear his name of heresy.

I'm not here to take a stance on religion (although I am not afraid to do that); I only bring up this history as an example of how hard it can be to accept a new scientific truth that goes against a current, entrenched belief system. The defective theory is deeply ingrained in AA and our culture. However, it doesn't have to be. If Bill Wilson were alive today, I'm certain he would not oppose modern scientific findings on alcohol. He wanted a cure for alcohol addiction more than anything. Unfortunately, Wilson founded AA at a time when humanity lacked the science to understand alcohol, and the organization has not updated their teachings to reflect new findings.

Even the Dalai Lama, the highest spiritual leader of Tibetan Buddhism, has famously said, "If science proves some belief of Buddhism wrong, then Buddhism would have to change."[9] I like to imagine Bill Wilson running into an AA meeting, jumping for joy and exclaiming in full voice:

It's not us! It's not us! We are not defective! It's the alcohol! It's addictive to anyone who consumes enough of it! There's no addictive allergy, gene, or personality!

We were unconscious and brainwashed the whole time we thought it was okay for people to drink alcohol! We can really be cured! Thank God! We will finally be completely free!

The majority of us who got addicted to alcohol have had childhood trauma. Therefore, I would like to share some of my story with you now. My childhood in rural Vermont was shattered at age eleven when my parents divorced. My trauma was accompanied by feelings of abandonment when my father moved to British Columbia and my mother moved to Boston. Around this time, I experienced the first of a series of depressions that I struggled with throughout my life.

Now, what vulnerable and brave soul would like to come up and share next?

DETOX TIMELINE: ONE YEAR ALCOHOL-FREE

You didn't believe me.

At the start of this book, I wrote, "You can do this. Trust me."

And here you are, a year into your alcohol-free journey. You feel better and look better. Your mind is clearer, and your wallet is heavier. Your cardiovascular system no longer experiences rebound stress, and your outer cortical brain areas continue to regain normal functioning. You no longer experience "hangxiety"; you now hardly remember what it feels like. Your risk of drinking again continues to drop.

But don't let your alcohol-free accomplishments go to your head. More precisely, don't let your alcohol-free accomplishments inflate your ego. Falling back into the Alcohol Matrix can happen even after years of being alcohol-free, so make sure you keep your consciousness (what I call being "fully awake") clean with daily meditation and affirmations.

When I was drinking—when I was stuck in ego-centered fear—I was always either less than or better than everyone I met: Stronger or weaker. Dominant or more subservient. Righteous or a more regular sinner. Better-looking or uglier. More athletic or clumsier. Smarter or dumber. Taller or shorter. The ego never stops comparing, which can invite intrusive thoughts into your head. There's an old saying: compare and despair.

A clear example of comparing consciousness is when I was a modeling extra on the movie set of *Jerry Maguire*, starring Tom Cruise.

The scene was in an office, and I was put in a UCLA jacket in a cubicle next to where director Cameron Crowe was set up for his main shot. He kept telling us this was the "fish scene": the most dramatic scene of the film, with the longest lines.

While we waited for Tom to come out of his trailer, I chatted with the attractive young lady in the cubicle next to me about the weather, and then we started talking about life in general. She was from Texas, and we talked about growing up as Okies and Texans and how different it was in Hollywood.

She was really smart, and we had a nice connection. I felt like she was interested in me and possibly wanted me to ask her out. At the time, I had lingerie models literally hanging on my back at photo shoots all day, so I thought, *I can probably get better.* But after about ten more minutes of great conversation, I was about to ask her out, when Tom suddenly came on the set. He performed his scene in a mystical, magical, mesmerizing way that I had never witnessed before. I was in a trance watching him perform with such passion and present-moment focus. Say what you will about his wacky religion, that man can act!

Toward the end of the scene, he scooped a fish out of the tank, put it in a bag, and asked about three hundred people in that huge "office," "Anyone going with me?"

The girl I had been talking to started to move, like she was thinking about getting up and possibly saying something. Meanwhile, Tom tried to get another office lady to come with him and had no luck.

"Okay, anybody else?" he asked.

Suddenly, my cute Texas sweetheart stood boldly and knocked a cup of coffee on herself. *Oh my god, no!* I thought, *She just ruined his perfect take!* Scooting out of my chair a little, I thought I could possibly reach out across the aisle and pull her back down into her chair. But it was too late.

Tom yelled out, "Dorothy Boyd, thank you!" He strode to her, and they exited together.

The two of them came back and everyone applauded as they made their way to Cameron. The three of them discussed how it went, and Cameron told Tom and his costar to take a break while he watched the film to see if they needed to do another take.

They didn't.

The Texas girl sat back down next to me. My eyes opened wide, and I was short of breath. I muscled out the words, "So you're the costar with Tom?"

She smiled at me. "Yeah."

I nodded my head and slinked back into my cubicle in total insecurity, feeling less than and fearful of her because she was so much wealthier and more famous than I was, and in total belief that there was no way she would ever go out with me.

I later found out that her name was Renée Zellweger. She had only been in small parts in movies like *Dazed and Confused* up to that point, so I had no idea who she was. By the way, you can't see me in the film, because the shots near Renée were all close up, so I didn't make the big silver screen.

Compare and despair!

I am sure Renée doesn't remember me at all—I didn't "have her at hello" like Tom did—but I want her and every woman to know that they are perfect unique expressions of consciousness. It took me over twenty years from the making of that film to fully realize that I am not better than or less than anyone else.

However much I exercise in a day, I make sure to sit down, be still, and close my eyes for the same amount of time. I like to sit in my car and meditate, either before or after a workout, but especially after my workouts, when my body and mind are calm and I can slip into a more deeply relaxed state. Car seats these days are incredibly comfortable, and you can position them for perfect posture for meditating!

Now, when I look at others who consume alcohol, I don't feel better than or less than them. I don't have any judgment, and I don't have any longing or jealousy either. I just slap my forehead and wonder, *How in the hell did I ever drink that stuff and pay a ton of money for it?*

Alcohol addiction is literally everywhere, as you've come to understand. But, like me, you've also come to realize, a year into your alcohol-free journey, that it no longer has anything to do with you.

CHAPTER 10

The Lie Alcohol Told Me:
"You Don't Have to Apologize for Anything"

The Truth I Figured Out:
I Have to Forgive Myself before Others Can Forgive Me

I wasted years on drinking, which caused nearly catastrophic damage, not only to me but to the people I love most in the world. Trapped in my addiction and held captive in the Alcohol Matrix, I didn't know what I didn't know. I was acting unconsciously and, more often than I like to admit, unconscionably. But, of course, I continued carrying on with my bad behavior and bad attitude, oblivious to the consequences looming over me, as sure as tomorrow's rising sun.

Because I wasn't yet awake, I still didn't realize I had anything to apologize for. Many, many transgressions, in fact. More than a year into being alcohol-free, I still wasn't able to apologize to the people I hurt the most. What was preventing me from doing so wasn't shame. Not exactly. What was stopping me from asking for forgiveness from others was the simple fact that I had yet to forgive myself.

My journey toward self-forgiveness was difficult. And, to be perfectly frank, a little weird, and a tad woo-woo, too. But let's be honest: is it any weirder than the thunder-throwing Zeus tattooed above my butt? Not really. Not as far as I'm concerned.

Ever since I was a teenager, I've had this reoccurring dream in which I fly around and teach other people how to fly. It always starts the same way. I'm in an immense room, a dimly lit library filled with thousands of books stacked on mahogany shelves. A bunch of kids are around me, waiting for me to take flight. I close my eyes, and after a minute or two of focus, my entire body begins to fill with light and starts to tingle. My feet gently rise off the wooden floor. Surprised, I lose focus and drop back down. I close my eyes and concentrate again on the tingling sensations in my hands, and up I go again, higher and higher. The other kids begin to jump up and down in excitement, yelling, "Look! He's doing it! He's flying!" I fly back down to them and begin teaching them. I tell them to close their eyes and focus inward until their bodies tingle. They lift off the ground and begin to fly around with me.

As an adult in my thirty-day treatment center, I had a one-hour Reiki healing session and right after that a rapid, deep breathwork session for another hour. It was two full hours of healing, torture, and, in my mind, trying to fly. (That dream again!) When the Reiki session began, I felt like I was a broken angel with a severely wounded throat and body, lying on the vast white marble floor of the Vatican, looking up as the Reiki therapist, a large angel with beautiful white wings, hovered over me. Emitting consciousness through her hands, she worked the broken parts of my body for nearly an hour. I left the Reiki experience feeling much better, but I was still stuck on the cold marble floor, unable to fly.

Five minutes later, I went over to the breathwork room with the same Reiki master and four other inpatients. When I began the hour-long, heavy and forceful deep breathing exercise under the Reiki master's guidance, I let my mind wander. It went immediately back into my childhood. I was a five-year-old experiencing the trauma of witnessing my father beat my mother. I found myself going back and forth from being a fallen angel on the Vatican floor to being a child in the kitchen with my family while my dad abused my mother.

As I went deeper into the breathwork, my angelic body on the floor of the Vatican began to heal, and I imagined I was able to fly a little. I flew up to a large empty wooden cross and became like Jesus being crucified, with massive stakes in my hands and feet. I kept going back and forth. I was screaming and crying as my three siblings and I watched my father beat my mother, and then suddenly I would be back on the cross, where I was in total agony as well.

The people in the room with me became my family. Darron was represented by another gay man in the room. There were three other women in the room besides the Reiki master, and one became my mother, while the other two became my two sisters. The Reiki master was still an angel doing healing work over us and making sure that we were safe. She was in all white, with enormous white angel wings. The suffering went on for a solid fifty minutes, back and forth from me being on the cross to watching my mother and father fighting.

Finally, I found my five-year-old face directly in front of my mom's bruised face. I calmly looked into her blood-soaked eyes and told her that we are all safe now and don't need to suffer anymore. I was released from the kitchen and flashed to being an angel who had now been healed. I ascended off the cross and flew around the Vatican rafters in Immortal Joy.

I told you it was a little out there, but there's a lesson here. This Reiki-and-deep-breathing-induced experience, laden with enough Catholic imagery to give even Martin Scorsese pause, helped me start to transform that punitive version of a god ready to smite me down that I have tattooed above my ass into a more beneficent one of unconditional love and total acceptance. "To understand everything," the Buddha said, "is to forgive everything." Following this experience, I forgave myself. I stopped wasting time feeling guilty about the years I squandered drinking alcohol. I no longer resented my alcohol-addicted past. I no longer felt any shame. Instead, I learned how to practice compassion and some long-overdue self-forgiveness.

Rather than letting myself off the hook, I accepted self-forgiveness as an essential part of moving on. Forgiving the self, as one study recently showed, is "an adaptive mechanism" to help people restore a positive sense of self and guard against the lingering, toxic effects of guilt, shame, and regret—all of which prevent us from moving forward without beating ourselves up over and over for our past poor behavior.[1] Self-forgiveness limits self-recrimination and self-condemnation—in their place, it opens up the opportunity to practice reaffirmation and, finally, self-acceptance. "Empirical evidence suggests that self-forgiveness is linked with high self-esteem, low neuroticism and low levels of anxiety and depression," the authors of the study wrote. "Similarly, it has been found to be positively linked with positive emotions, and with a lack of shame. Numerous studies have consistently demon[s]trated that self-forgiveness has a positive impact on overall well-being. For instance, when people self-forgive their feelings, attitudes and beliefs toward the self become more positive and this in turn leads to lower levels of depressive affect."[2]

First and foremost, learning to forgive myself allowed me to protect myself against lingering feelings of guilt and regret. This afforded me the room to figure out how to accept myself, faults and all, and, over time, learn to love myself.

Like me, you probably didn't consciously know what you were doing when you first started drinking, so have compassion for your past 1.0 version of yourself who didn't know the facts about alcohol. From a young age, you watched and listened to countless ads promoting alcohol. You consumed an addictive toxin because you grew up watching virtually every adult around you do the same. Forgive yourself for being human, for not being able to consciously see through our collective illusion that says alcohol benefits us, and for being born into a world that is currently addicted to alcohol. Forgive yourself for getting addicted to a liquid that you were told was only addictive to certain "defective" people.

At the same time, remember you were the one who took every drink of alcohol you've ever had. As the Tibetan Buddhist scholar Lama Zopa Rinpoche teaches, "You are responsible for your own problems just as you're responsible for your own liberation and enlightenment." You must also forgive yourself for any wrongful behaviors caused by alcohol, for ways you mistreated your family and friends while under the influence, for events you never showed up to, for responsibilities you didn't follow through on, and for promises you broke. You aren't a bad person. But alcohol influenced you to make bad decisions. Rather than plaguing yourself with guilt over these mistakes, remind yourself that you're better now that alcohol isn't in your life. Your alcohol-addicted past is over. You are not your past. You are so much more than any addiction. You deserve forgiveness because you've proven—to yourself and to others—that you are a changed person with much higher consciousness than before. As the 2.0 version of yourself, you now treat others in a kind and considerate way.

To drive these points home, I like to say this mantra by Mark Santiago—I even took a photo of it and used it as my phone wallpaper for a while:

I am responsible . . .

I am responsible for the life I live. It is no one else's responsibility but my own.

I am responsible for all the good and all the bad.

I am responsible for who I allow into my life.

I am responsible for how I show up.

I am responsible for my wins and my losses.

I am responsible for my thoughts and my decisions.

And because I'm responsible . . . I can CHOOSE the kind of life I want.

Life doesn't happen to me . . . I happen to life.

I choose to be present.

I choose to love.

I choose to be intimate.

I choose to be joyful.

I choose to be EMPOWERED . . .
and no one can take that from me without my permission.

After I did a thirty-day meditation/yoga retreat in Southeast Asia, I vowed to be in silence for a minimum of a month. Each week at the retreat, we did a day of silence, and I realized through those days and through our two hours a day of silent meditations and two hours a day of silent yoga that in my normal life I spoke way too much and tried to control everything and everyone by speaking. After the retreat, I decided to continue my vow of silence back in my normal California life. In total, I ended up not speaking for a full sixty days. When I was finally ready to break my silence, the first thing I did was ask my then-wife and my children for forgiveness. My vocal cords struggled to voice my remorse. I could hardly speak. Finally mustering up the words I'd held in for so long, I sounded like a thirteen-year-old boy going through puberty. But I spoke and finally expressed my deep remorse. I apologized to my estranged wife for traumatizing her and violating her. And I told her that her anger in response to my actions forced me to grow in ways I never thought possible. I expressed gratitude for her strength and righteousness. I told my daughters how much I loved them and that I never meant to hurt them in any way. I got on one knee, looked them both in the eyes, and said that I was doing everything I knew how to get better and that I would make it all up to them, and then some, once I healed. I thanked them for their support and patience with me during such a difficult time of my life.

You may need to say "I am sorry" to a lot of people you hurt along the agonizing path of alcohol addiction. Just because you were unconscious in the past, do not ever excuse yourself by not taking responsibility for your actions. Forgive yourself, but never excuse. You hurt a lot of people. Accept it. Know it. Go into it and feel all of the pain that you caused. Then *apologize*!

Do not be afraid to apologize and mend those relationships.

I have never met a person who didn't respond well to a sincere apology. The people in your life to whom you will apologize miss the way you were before alcohol, and they are going to be ecstatic that you're back, even if your relationship takes a different shape.

TURNING WINE INTO WATER

There was one time when I wouldn't apologize for my behavior.

I was at an otherwise lovely dinner at my in-laws' house. My father-in-law, the kindest, most compassionate, and most non-judgmental man I have ever been around, was drinking wine. My oldest daughter, who was six at the time, asked him, "Papa, why do you drink wine?"

You could see Papa's eyes widen a bit as he choked down his sip of red wine. He set his glass down, paused for a minute, and said, "Well, it makes my food taste better."

The other adults at the table were relieved to get through this question and move on to how our local sports team played and what the best part of the day was for each of us. Not me, though. No way, no how. I am alcohol-free, and my girls are *not* going to listen to this unscientific hogwash being spewed out by a man I love and respect so much.

My ex-wife asked my four-year-old how her day was, but I put my condescending, *I am more educated than you* finger up and said, "One second, please." Then I turned to my two daughters. "Girls, did you know that there is thirteen percent alcohol in wine, and science has proven to us that alcohol deadens and numbs everything it touches? This means that when you drink a liquid with alcohol in it, like beer or wine with dinner, your taste buds get deadened and go numb."

My intelligent four-year-old turned to my ex-wife and asked, "What is numb?" My ex-wife calmly shook her head. She glared at me with the look that a husband knows deep inside the bowels of his soul says: *I cannot believe you are doing this right now.* But did that stop my all-knowing, all-powerful, scientific ego from continuing on? Haha! Don't be ridiculous.

My ego still had full control of me at this point, and I was in it to win it. Ironically, I was lost in my *educated* thought! Defeat the Alcohol Matrix at all costs!

"So, girls," I continued, "when Papa says he likes to drink wine because it makes his food taste better, science says it actually numbs, which means it takes away or lowers, your taste buds' ability to taste by about thirty percent. If you really want to taste your food fully at a hundred percent, then you don't want to drink anything with alcohol in it before or while you eat."

"What are taste buds?" my four-year-old asked.

I was about to go into my professorial lecture on this important topic, but I got another look from my ex-wife, and this time it was not the *Really?* look—it was the *You're dead if you do not stop right now* look. Even her light hazel eyes turned red when she said it! That look finally hit home. I felt very unwelcome and got up from the dinner table to go proudly pour myself some kombucha in the kitchen, having slain the Alcohol Matrix monster and, unfortunately, my father-in-law in the battle.

Since apologizing to my ex-wife and daughters, I have apologized to everyone I can think of whom I ever harmed while I was addicted to alcohol. I thought about apologizing for this one too, but you know what? The Alcohol Matrix gets to spew its millions of lies all over the world every day. It has never apologized once. So, sorry, not sorry, Dad!

When I finally started to forgive myself and others, I learned how to break free of remorse, shame, guilt, and self-pity. I loved myself for making it through my addiction. As the St. Francis prayer says, "It is by forgiving that one is forgiven. It is by dying that one awakens to eternal life." I took these words to heart and offered compassion to the people in my life who hurt me most.

Before my dad died of esophageal cancer, he and I started to talk more. Or at least talk more honestly with one another. During one of our heart-to-hearts, I told him that I forgave him. I forgave him for abusing my mom, psychically and emotionally. I forgave him for traumatizing me and my siblings. Even though he never fully apologized for either. Or anything else. Remember the story I told you about when Dad busted into our house, clad in his cowboy boots, and kicked our living room table in a rage? When he launched the glass of iced tea to the ceiling?

What I didn't tell you was Darron was trying to hide in the garage. When my dad ran out of the house through the garage to escape the cops, Darron watched him go. Then he yelled to the cop, hot in pursuit, "He's going to the back gate!" My dad yelled back, *"My own son!"* He was disgusted with Darron for betraying him.

"Now just sit with that a minute," Darron told me once. "Do you know how big an asshole you have to be to get upset and disgusted with your ten-year-old child, whose house you've just busted into, whose mother and guest you've assaulted, and whose living room table you've kicked to the ceiling? Now how big of an asshole do you have to be not to apologize the next day, or ever, and to continue to remind that child how he told the cops on you and how ashamed you were of him?"

My dad acknowledged my forgiveness, then he and I never spoke of it again. Just like so many people who die of alcohol addiction or alcohol-related illnesses, he didn't know what he didn't know. Because of his inability to be vulnerable, my dad remained what we call a dry drunk (more on this in the next chapter). He wasn't able to access certain parts of himself, though I am happy to know he found some kind of inner peace later in life. He kept a quote in his room, a quote from the poet Henry Wadsworth Longfellow: "If we could read the secret history of our enemies, we should find in each man's life sorrow and suffering enough to disarm all hostility." When my dad died, I read it at his funeral.

Since I stopped drinking, I have learned to live fully and freely in the present moment, simply as I am. Doing so has opened me up in ways I never thought possible. I no longer resent the people who hurt or betrayed me. I am aware of their secret histories, and I am conscious of their sorrow and their suffering, which disarms my hostility. I am now transforming my consciousness.

Forgiveness isn't reserved for people of faith, or a specific religion. A professor at the University Wisconsin–Madison notes how forgiveness improves a person's mental and physical health. "Forgiveness really isn't about you," says Robert Enright, an expert in forgiveness science in the school's Department of Education Psychology. "It's for the other person, but you reap the benefits."[3] Another study across five countries showed that when forgiveness is taught, practiced, and achieved, the result is better mental and overall well-being, most notably lowering depression and decreasing symptoms of anxiety.[4]

Letting go and moving on is good for you. It's another step in your lifelong journey of being awake and alcohol-free. Yes, we have to own up to our past behavior. But, at the same time, we get to own our way forward.

My own personal way forward is through spiritual retreats and deepening my consciousness. I own a gorgeous, historic waterfront lodge on Table Rock Lake in Eureka Springs, Arkansas. Because of the area's mountainous landscape, that part of the country is known as "America's Little Switzerland." The town and lodge are built on ground full of crystals, and natural water springs cascade around them. It is a spot with some of the most peaceful and serene energy in the world. It's not a coincidence that Eureka is also affectionately called "Eufreaka," thanks to its open, fun, social vibe and rainbow flag–waving locals. And let me tell you, I proudly fly that "Eufreaka," flag these days! In fact, I actually convinced the founder of Hariharalaya in Cambodia, my favorite retreat center in the world, to replicate the center at my lodge. From my place, you can look out over the lake. In the distance is a charming one-lane yellow wooden bridge. Whenever I feel myself drifting or getting lost in intrusive thoughts, I like to visualize this yellow bridge: a path home, back to myself.

Since my awakening from alcohol, I've experienced many moments that have allowed me to return home, back to myself.

This is where I started to measure the time I've gained in my real life in terms of years, not just weeks or months. At this point I've been able to spend more real, present-moment hours with those I love and be creative in writing in this book, instead of spending it with a toxic liquid.

I recently had a conversation with a kind waiter at a high-end restaurant. He had approached me with a white towel on his arm and a glass of white wine on a silver tray, proudly telling me, "This Sauvignon Blanc pairs perfectly with the goat cheese and fig appetizer you are having."

"No, thank you," I replied.

"But it comes with the appetizer for free."

"No, thank you, I don't drink cancer juice."

"Cancer juice?"

"Yes, scientists have proven for a one hundred percent fact that ethanol causes cancer."

"Ethanol?"

"Yes, ethanol is the exact same thing as alcohol; it just has two different names."

"I thought ethanol was a type of gasoline?"

"It is, and that is why when people consume it on a regular basis, it causes cancer and a lot of other diseases. There is about thirteen percent gasoline in that glass you're holding."

"Wow. You know a lot about alcohol."

"Your body knows infinitely more about alcohol than I ever will. Listen to it. But again, thank you for the offer. May I have an Arnold Palmer, please?"

From two years onward, improvements are less likely to feel dramatic. You've experienced the extra money. You've reclaimed the extra time. You've felt the wonderful health benefits, like living at a higher level of consciousness, increased physical strength, lower body fat, and deeper sleep. Your children want to be around you more. You've made new friends, rebuilt your family ties, boosted your mood, and found better ways to enjoy life. You have tremendously increased your odds of living longer and are experiencing more joy. Your appreciation for your new lifestyle is peaking, and you'll be able to ride that high plateau for as long as you stay away from the toxic, impotence-causing liquid that held you down for so long.

You have been working on any underlying psychological issues through meetings, counselors, sponsors, research, meditation, and exercise. You are shining the light of consciousness on all fears and insecurities. They are dissolving rapidly, and you are beginning to feel your true, joyous, timeless self come out more each day.

You witness the Alcohol Matrix, but you're no longer a part of it or affected by it. You are awake.

As Annie Grace says, once we have our awakening, we need to pay it forward. It is now your turn to become the next messenger. Please join the Alcohol-Free Revolution with me today, right now. One by one, we can collectively dissolve Big Alcohol advertising and the Alcohol Matrix monster together. I can assure you that it will be one of the most rewarding ventures of your life and that you will never regret it. We are the AFR!

Here are some ways you can join the revolution:

- Send loving, supportive emails to the friends or loved ones who you think are most ready to wake up from the Alcohol Matrix.

- Go to your local bookstore and find your favorite alcohol-awakening book. (It doesn't have to be this one!)

Send print or e-books to at least three people you know who have been affected by the Alcohol Matrix.

- Get one more copy of your favorite alcohol-awakening book and donate it to your local library.

- Talk honestly to the kids in your life, especially teenagers, about the Alcohol Matrix.

- Have fun starting conversations with total strangers, like bartenders and servers, about ethanol.

- To get free tips, coaching, resources, and more, join my community, the Alcohol-Free Revolution, at WeAretheAFR.org, or simply scan the QR code below.

CHAPTER 11

The Lie Alcohol Told Me:
"You Can Never Escape the Alcohol Matrix"

The Truth I Figured Out:
I Can Live in a Joyous, Alcohol-Free Consciousness

It is time for me to be unapologetically spiritual.

Don't worry, I'll keep it light. In case you haven't noticed, my three traveling companions are Jesus, Buddha, and Eckhart Tolle. Even though I practice Buddhist meditation, I am a lot like Ricky Bobby in the movie *Talladega Nights*. In one scene, Ricky Bobby tells his wife that he likes to say the dinner prayer to a Christmas baby Jesus. "When you say grace, you can say it to grown-up Jesus, or teenage Jesus, or bearded Jesus, or whoever you want." Or how about Ricky's sidekick, Cal Naughton Jr., who says, "I like to picture Jesus in a tuxedo T-shirt, cuz it says, like, I want to be formal, but I'm here to party, too."

That's me, basically: a tuxedo T-shirt–wearing Jesus, mixed with a little potbellied Buddha—though after all these years living alcohol-free, my abs are thankfully more like Jesus' washboard midsection than Buddha's pronounced paunch!

While we're on the subject of Buddha, let's talk about the

Buddhist term *nirvana*. It means a transcendent state in which there is neither suffering nor lust for anything or anyone, and you are released from the effects of karma and the cycle of death and rebirth. It is the ultimate realization of Buddhism. This is what it's been like for me to awaken out of the Alcohol Matrix. You realize there is never again a need to drink alcohol. You have no suffering or lust over alcohol at all. It becomes a nonissue. There is no more suffering because there is no more lusting for a substance that you know at the deepest level is addictive and toxic.

Alcohol-free nirvana is not some magical, mystical unicorn experience that only a select few can have. It is wide open and available to everyone. All you have to do is get your entire consciousness to agree that alcohol is bad for you. That is it. Once the unconscious part of your mind has been completely unbrainwashed to agree with your conscious mind that alcohol is ethanol and ethanol is an addictive, rotten liquid that no one should consume (just like no one should inhale cigarettes), you will reach alcohol-free nirvana. You will have no desire to consume a substance that is poisonous.

But quitting alcohol is just the start. I deeply respect AA cofounder Bill Wilson's observation that even after some addicts had become alcohol-free, their pattern of selfish and self-destructive behavior of not being vulnerable, not apologizing, blaming and shaming others, playing the victim role, or acting holier than thou stayed the same as when they were drinking. The phrase he coined for this is a "dry drunk." Bill knew that the true objective of AA was not simply to help people to no longer drink, but also to make their lives better by getting to the core of any personal anxiety and pain.

Below are significant indicators that you might be a dry drunk. I include this term and self-reflection not to cause self-judgment or self-condemnation but instead to assist you in knowing whether there is more healing to be done. I engaged in virtually all of these behaviors the year after I stopped drinking, believe me.

After becoming alcohol-free, if you begin to have feelings of resentment or anger, that is a major sign that you are a dry drunk. When you believe in any way that you are a victim of your life situation or others are against you, that is being a dry drunk. Let's dig a little deeper:

- Do you keep trying to be the center of attention (even though you're not drinking) in a bar full of drunks who are pretending to listen to you and your loud ego grasping for validation and approval? Dry drunk.

- Does your mood go from happiness to sadness? Dry drunk (or possibly mental health issues if it is extreme, so get professional help if this happens).

- Do you believe that being alcohol-free is boring? Dry drunk.

- Do you have anger and resentment toward family and friends who intervened in your addictive drinking? Dry drunk.

- Do you have a hard time being vulnerable and communicating honestly and openly with others? Dry drunk.

- Are you afraid that you cannot change? Dry drunk.

- Do you refuse to accept others' constructive criticism of you? Dry drunk.

- Do you still crave a drink? Dry drunk.

Up until this point, you have self-medicated your high-functioning, overthinking mind with a toxin for so many years. It is time to drop the addictive bottle, get a sleeping mask and some earplugs, go to a quiet space, sit down, close your eyes, and let silence truly heal your incessantly thinking mind.

MEDITATION AS MEDICINE

I strongly believe that meditation is an invaluable tool for healing. As Jerry Seinfeld once said, meditation and weight training "could solve just about anyone's life." Extensive research has proved that meditation is one of the most powerful tools to aid in your recovery (and life in general). I meditate daily, sometimes more than an hour at a time, and I still have egotistical thoughts that bubble up and try to hijack me: *Am I worthy? Am I enough? Am I ugly? Do people like me? Am I better than them or less than them? Am I smart? Can I write? Please love me!*

A big reason why high-functioning addicts (like I was) drink alcohol is to alleviate and control our incessant thinking and future-planning egos. Meditation helps you control that false ego thinking and keeps you calm in a natural, peaceful, high-consciousness way, without putting any addictive poison into your body. You will go above thought, instead of numbing down and suppressing thought. You will come out of your meditations feeling centered and peaceful. While in meditation, you go beyond ego. Your mind is cleansed with each meditation, even when you feel, think, see, hear, or taste absolutely nothing. A mantra I say right before I meditate is, "In silence I receive." Meditation is an invisible, silent, and healing medication.

With your heightened focus, awareness, and mood, you'll be able to gain peace of mind. You will have a newfound clarity to tackle any obstacle life throws at you. Say and use this Pema Chödrön mantra in your meditations: "You are the sky, everything else is just the weather." Storms will come and go. No matter the severity of the storm or how long it is in you, it will pass.

Another important step in healing is to face yourself head-on and deal with any and all of your psychological problems. You must get to the root of the pain, fear, and anxiety that you covered for so many years by drinking. The incredible news is that by removing alcohol, your true-self journey can now begin. But do not believe that it will be easy. By removing your very temporary "pain medication," you are going to literally feel everything!

Do not shy away from any anxiety or pain that surfaces after you become alcohol-free. The Sufi poet Rumi wrote, "These pains you feel are messengers. Listen to them." Lean into all of the pain and anxiety. Where is it truly coming from? What happened to you as a child or as a teenager? To explore this issue, here are some questions to consider:

- Who or what hurt you?
- Were you ignored because one or both of your parents were workaholics?
- Did your parents divorce?
- Were one or both of your parents addicts?
- Have they ever shown signs of narcissism, bipolar disorder, depression, codependency, or an eating disorder?
- Do you live in fear of not having enough money?
- Were you sexually abused?
- Do you have a fear of being alone?
- Do you have a deep unconscious fear of death and being banished and abandoned by the universe, like I used to have?

Until you dive deeply into your past pain/trauma and realize its higher purpose and meaning in your life, you will not heal it completely.

During my monthlong meditation and yoga retreat in Southeast Asia, I felt confident in my ability to overcome my addiction to alcohol. But I had just signed my divorce papers, so I wanted to step away from the situation and center myself, in the hope of maintaining some much-needed balance. Even halfway around the world, however, I struggled to distance myself from my problems. I was having a hard time remaining present. I watched retreatant after retreatant express their deepest vulnerabilities and deepest hurts. And all I could do was hold back.

Until one morning.

While I was on the retreat, I was also completing a workbook, *Calling in "the One"* by the enlightened breakup guru Katherine Woodward Thomas. At the same time, I was also participating in a weekly community circle, where we shared our stories and thoughts with the group. Before each circle, we had to read a poem the night before. During the circle, we'd go around and share what resonated most with us about the poem. For this particular circle, we were asked to read a poem by Hafiz, a Sufi mystic, called "Now Is the Time." I include part of it here:

> Now is the time to know
>
> That all that you do is sacred.
>
> Now, why not consider
>
> A lasting truce with yourself and God.
>
> Now is the time to understand
>
> That all your ideas of right and wrong
>
> Were just a child's training wheels

To be laid aside

When you can finally live

With veracity

And love.

As instructed, I read the poem the night before the community sharing circle. And, man, did that poem hit me right between the eyes. I was up all night. Compassion for myself and all others at the retreat opened like a lotus flower in the sun. Loving awareness flooded through me. I couldn't wait for the sharing circle to start. I had to get what was inside of me out. I needed to release it. On every other occasion, I would choose to sit away from the leader of the circle so I wouldn't have to speak right away. This time I got there early and purposely sat right next to the leader, ready to speak first.

As I mentioned, a few of the others had been incredibly vulnerable, brave, and humble enough to share their past traumas or transgressions committed against them, or that they themselves had committed.

When I volunteered to speak, I told the group that poem initially reminded me of the times in my life when things went really well. Like my wedding day, when my kids were born, and every other joyous experience in life. Those were my sacred moments. But then I turned and began putting that idea on my lowest moments of life: watching my dad beat my mother, the four times I acted out against my ex-wife, and the final year of my drinking.

I began speaking to the group.

"Due to watching my father beat my mother and having him abandon me, I unconsciously grasped for attention, validation, and love from alcohol and people my whole life. I became unconsciously addicted to trying to get others to love me. While on an extremely drunk golf trip with a bunch of other men, I sent a text proposing sex to an Uber driver. On the same golf trip, I went to the back room of a strip club. About six months later, on a similar drunk golf trip, we all went to another strip club and went to the back rooms again. A month after that, I went to a massage parlor for sex and wasn't even that drunk when I did it. That was acting more out of my love addiction than alcohol addiction. I did all of this while my beautiful ex-wife was at home with our small children. This is what caused her to separate from me over a year ago.

"These moments carry so much anger, resentment, shame, and guilt. I now refer to them as my sacred wound moments. They have made me who and what I am today. Without them, I would not have gained much wisdom at all. With them, I have become vulnerable, patient, kind, a good listener, forgiving, compassionate, and, most of all, they have made me humble. All of the good things in me have been activated because of those horrible sacred wound moments. I would have never had the understanding, insight, or motivation to work on a book for over two years in an attempt to help others with addictions."

I paused and looked around the circle. As I spoke, I looked into the eyes of each person around me.

"My friend from Canada, you were so humble and open to tell us that five years ago you were dead inside from doing so many drugs, and now you are a leader in Narcotics Anonymous who speaks to thousands of prison inmates. It is clear to me now that all of the times you were doing drugs were sacred.

"My friend from France, you were so vulnerable and brave to tell us all that you were raped at the age of fifteen. I can now see that out of this dreadful sacred moment, you had the motivation and desire to help others so much that you became a clinical psychologist.

"My friend from Cambodia, your baby girl died in your arms moments after being born. Having already had your present moment awakening, due to all of your sacred wound moments in your life, you were able to be completely present for her and say mantras and prayers to her while she took her first and few last breaths. You understood completely and fully accepted her death right then and there. As you said, you knew, then and now, that 'everything is divine timing, and I cannot possibly fathom what that is; I just have to get out of the way.'"

Part of becoming alcohol-free is to learn from all of our sacred wound moments. Ask yourself what you did that is still causing you guilt or shame. Once again, go into the exact scene and moment, and visualize it as intensely as you can. What are the smells and sounds; who is there? See yourself clearly doing whatever it was that you did.

Work intensely within yourself (and with a professional, if needed) to go back to the exact moments of your most traumatic/painful experience in your youth. Who and/or what is there with you? What are the smells? What can you hear? Is there screaming? Who do you have anger toward? Who do you still resent for what they did to you? Face your trauma, pain, and fear, once and for all. We have all been hurt.

Now ask yourself what your life would be like without these sacred wounds? Would you be humble? Would you have compassion and empathy for others? Would you want to help others? Now is the time for you to deeply realize that every thought and every action you have ever had or done or that has happened to you is sacred. Realize the impossibility that there is anything but grace. You are not alone. You have never been alone. You will never walk alone.

If you want to end a lot of suffering and find your true self-acceptance, I highly recommend doing the *Calling in "the One"* book/workbook. In it, Thomas created a practice that sets the intention for receiving the love of your life. I have altered it here for setting a clear intention of living alcohol-free.

Please take out a piece of paper and a pen (not your phone). Think deeply, and be crystal clear about what it is you want and when you want it, and write it down by hand. For example: "My intention is that I will not have any cravings to drink alcohol by _____ [fill in date]. At that time, it will even make me feel a little bit sick if I do think about drinking it."

Complete these sentences:

- My intention is:
- I am in integrity with this future when I:
- I am out of integrity with this future when I:
- By living alcohol-free, I desire to experience:
- To generate this experience now, I can:
- Being alcohol-free, I desire to create:
- To create this now, I can:

Put your completed work somewhere you will see it often, and read it to yourself when you do see it.

Along my journey, one important question I learned to ask myself is: *Am I going to react out of love, or am I going to react out of fear?* That choice is, always has been, and always will be yours and yours alone. You will create your life out of your reactions.

As hard as it may seem when you begin to do this, try to choose to love everything and everyone all the time. Even, and especially, horrible, angry, mean, rude, obnoxious, impatient, and self-righteous people. In these moments, ask: "What would love do?"

The same goes for when these egoic issues arise in yourself. What would love do with yourself when you are feeling horrible, angry, mean, rude, obnoxious, impatient, and self-righteous? Love yourself when you feel these shadows in you. Choose to love yourself first and foremost. All of yourself, just as you are, even in the painful, fearful times of low-level ego consciousness. Then you will be able to love others the same way when they, too, are acting out of fear and need love most.

The most important spiritual lesson I learned along my journey is that consciousness comes from simply waking up to that fact, not from any book or lesson. The key is to look deep within yourself and remember: wake up. You were lost in a low-level consciousness dream governed by ego and fear for a very long time. Now, at this very moment, not some time in the future, you can wake up completely and never suffer from that false, separate, small-minded world again because you now realize fully that it is not who or what you are.

Dear reader, you are so much more than any addiction. You are not defective. Please awaken fully to the fact that no matter how painful your past has been, the present moment is all there is, all there ever has been, or ever will be. I urge you to stay out of your fearful, judging, ant-mind consciousness, stay out of the past and future, and reside in the eternal present moment.

CONCLUSION
Staying Alcohol-Free

I want to leave you with some tips as you start your new conscious life.

In the beginning of being alcohol-free, you will feel a strong desire to explain yourself to others. That's okay, but there's no need for explanation. Strangers, friends, and advertisements in the Alcohol Matrix can say whatever they want, and it won't change the truth you know about ethanol. Once you have fully realized that you never have to drink alcohol again, you can easily say, "No, thank you," as you pour yourself a delicious nonethanol drink.

You will be able to go to all the parties, clubs, and bars you want (if you want), and there will not be a single bottle of alcohol that will have any power over you. "I just feel a lot better when I don't drink" will flow from your mouth. Why would you drink something that is going to make you sick or even kill you? You know you're over it. You're fully awake. No one can or will ever be able to influence you to drink ever again.

Visualization is a key tool to help you navigate any events where ethanol is flowing. Now that you are awake and out of the illusion of the alcohol matrix (notice it is not capitalized anymore), you will need to use the power of your consciousness when you are surrounded by people who are still in it.

For example, if you are going to a social event, start from the beginning and visualize how you will get there (drive, Uber, walk) and who will go with you. Close your eyes and take a few deep breaths. See in your mind who is there once you arrive. Get detailed. What is the lighting like? What music is playing? Are there any smells?

Go through the room(s) and see if there is anyone there who triggers any anxiety. Who might be challenging to talk to? Is it someone specific, or a general kind of person (like a belligerent, obnoxious drunk)? Have a plan for interacting with them. Do you say hi? Do you speak with them? Is it okay if you don't talk to them? If you must have a conversation, then what will you say?

Do they ask you, "Why don't you drink anymore?" Actually, say out loud a few times, "I just feel a lot better when I don't drink." Then visualize yourself leaving it at that. It just creates unnecessary awkwardness if you keep explaining or say anything else about it when you are a rookie at being alcohol-free.

Ninety-five percent of the time, the person asking will accept your answer and move on. The other 5 percent of the time, the person who keeps asking why you don't drink is likely doing so because they are curious about your power over alcohol and want to learn from you. Feel them out, and if you want to share, go for it. If you ever feel like you're being attacked or pressured in any way, just know that no matter what they say, you have *all* the power compared with anyone who is sipping, or in the loud-mouth drunk's case, chugging down poison.

The most important part of this visualization is how to get out of the conversation if you're feeling any anxiety. I personally have to pee about every hour when I am in social situations, as I like to have a glass of sparkling water in my hands and drink a lot of it, so going to the bathroom is my "exit conversation." Most of the time it is the truth! "Good talking to you, I gotta run to the bathroom, but we'll catch up later."

What is your "exit conversation" statement? Know it and practice it. When I first started dating my ex-wife, she told me she couldn't get out of conversations with guys who were hitting on her, so we practiced her exit together. She would extend her hand to shake wannabe-Romeo's hand and say, "It was nice talking with you. I have to get back to my friends now." She said the best part was physically extending her hand when she wanted to be out of the conversation. It made the rest of her body commit to the escape. There are a lot of different exit strategies, so come up with one that is comfortable for you, visualize it, practice it, and say it out loud.

Don't drag out an exit. People think they are being good friends and hosts by trying to get you to stay. They think they are showing you how much they like you and want you there. This is true for them, and there's nothing wrong with it, but it is not what you need in your first few parties after awakening, or if you are ever feeling uncomfortable at a party in any way.

The absolute best way to definitively exit a party is to *simply leave*. Just walk out the door. This is why you need an exit plan, and the most important part of that plan is how you get home. Is it Uber, or will you drive yourself, walk, or ride a bike? See it. Know your exact way to go home before you get to the party. If you ever feel anxiety or the need to leave, *just go*. No need to say goodbye to anyone. Just walk right out in total silence. You can text anyone you need to later, if necessary. They will understand, and most of the time they are so busy in their own party world that they don't even notice.

When you are visualizing, you have absolutely no reason to envision negative scenarios or fantasies. Stay away from making up future scenes that end poorly. It is very healthy to be thinking clearly and planning in the present moment about tomorrow's party, where there will most likely be a lot of people drinking. However, after you plan your time of arrival, what you will wear, and how you will get there, if you then continue into a negative fantasy where you imagine yourself being uncomfortable, shy, self-conscious, not as good as the other people, and having less fun since they are drinking and you are not, that negates the value of your visualization. You will also make your negative fantasies become real if you visualize them enough. Watch all of your thoughts and future fantasies very closely and make sure they are coming from a place of no fear and all love. You create your future in the present moment with all of your thoughts and fantasies, both negative and positive.

The best thing to do is just plan your event in your mind, and then get back into the present moment with whatever you are actually doing. But if you are going to fantasize about a future event, be sure to imagine positive things. See yourself having fun, being social, laughing, dancing, and being as good as (not better than or less than) anyone else. Then come back to the present moment and get out of the future completely.

You create what you strive for and imagine. Strive for and imagine yourself living a real life being alcohol-free. Imagine having a blast with your friends, family, and society in general. Imagine having a bottle of water or nonalcoholic drink in your hand and dancing like no one is watching when there is great music. Imagine being totally at peace around anyone and everyone without the desire to put alcohol in your healthy body.

CONCLUSION

Imagine the liberation you will always feel when you're no longer in the alcohol matrix, affected by Big Alcohol advertising, or swayed by peer pressure to drink. Imagine the pure freedom you will feel when you no longer have any cognitive dissonance to justify your drinking habits. Imagine the earnest feeling of contentment and peace that comes from enjoying an alcohol-free life.

AFTERWORD
Where I Am Now: An Invitation

After I wrote this book, my ex-wife called me on her birthday to let me know she had filed for divorce. A week later, on Valentine's Day, she emailed me the divorce papers to sign. As you can clearly see, she's not angry with me at all!

The only reason I can make light of these events is because, thanks to the work I've done, I no longer have a fear of abandonment. Let me explain. My alcohol-free journey has been multi-faceted, and one aspect of this wild ride has been a willingness to get unapologetically spiritual. As I've already shared, I've been on many spiritual retreats and have allowed myself to go places emotionally and mentally that I'd never been before or even dreamed of. I'd like to give you a sense of what that has looked like for me, how freeing it has been, and to invite you to join me there. This might look very different from what your journey has looked like, and my beliefs may differ from yours, but I know there is value in sharing what I have learned by embracing my most "spiritual" self.

I've spent years going deep on my fear of abandonment and have learned a lot from the great Pema Chödrön, the first fully ordained Tibetan Buddhist female American. She writes: "All anxiety, all dissatisfaction, all the reasons for hoping that our experience could be different are rooted in our fear of death." In my understanding, Chödrön is referring to fear of abandonment—something we all experience whether we realize it or not. What I've also learned is that the only cure for this core fear is to awaken fully to the fact that at our most true essence we are eternal joy and therefore we can never be abandoned. But don't take my word for it. Let's hear from my three homies once again.

Buddha said, "A wise man, recognizing that the world is but an illusion, does not act as if it is real, so he escapes the suffering." My take: All external things die. See through the illusion that they are real, and you will find true peace.

As Jesus said, "In me you may have peace. In this world you will have trouble. But take heart! I have overcome the world." My read: overcome all worldly things and know deeply, as Jesus did, that all physical forms—the past, and the future—are illusions.

At a live talk I attended in Los Angeles, Eckhart Tolle described how our mindset can change when we realize the universe as we see it is an illusion. With this realization, we don't take everything so seriously. We are able to live with less stress, fear, conflict, and suffering.

This is not some new age thinking or airy-fairy spirituality (and if it is, then Jesus and Buddha were both new age, airy-fairy spiritual thinkers as well!). Here's how it looks to me in my newfound perspective: You are Christ consciousness, Buddha consciousness, eternal life, timeless, the unmanifested. Jesus said, "Is it not written in your Law, 'I have said you are gods?'"

Jesus was quoting the Old Testament, where God said, "Ye are gods; and all of you children of the Most High." He did not say anything like, "You might be a god," or "Some people are gods." "Ye" means you. *You* are a god. We are all gods. Listen, whatever your religious beliefs are is 100 percent cool with me. Just please hear my overall message: *Stop playing so small! Alcohol has zero power over you!*

I am also excited to share that I am opening a Hariharalaya USA in Eureka Springs, Arkansas, and I would love to see you there. We'll be hosting all-inclusive retreats (meditation courses, yoga classes, workshops, Reiki, massage, breathwork, digital detox, and healthy meals). To keep this experience affordable to all, the fee at Hari USA will be a fraction of the cost typically incurred at comparable retreats. There will be weeklong programs and thirty-day retreats. Although you can shed your cocoon in one week, I do believe that for a full metamorphosis to occur and to be able to fly, thirty days is the key.

To keep it intimate, we'll have about fifteen rooms and host about 180 people per year. The expected opening date is isn't set yet, but you can join Skool on the AFR website (www.WeAretheAFR.org) to stay updated on its opening. Until Hari USA is manifested, I encourage you to consider a trip to Cambodia and go directly to the mothership, as I have. If the Hariharalaya mothership can help transform an angry, fearful, anxiety-ridden, depressed, fighting, controlling, loudmouthed, arrogant guy like I was into a gentle, flying, loving white butterfly, then I am certain it will help you, too.

Finally, I want to share with you the most recent experience I had at Hariharalaya. I call it *The Elephant and the Butterfly*. Yeah, it's gonna get a little weird, so cut me some slack if you can. Here goes:

Once a week we would have a two-hour guided shamanic journey. We would all lie down on our yoga mats on our backs in a circle, with our heads pointed into the circle. There were no psychedelics ever used, only sound. We would also have a weekly one-hour evening dance. I chose to wear a blackout mask over my eyes the whole time I was dancing.

On the shamanic journeys, where I would often go into a liberating, dreamlike state, I got to hang out with my spirit animal—a white butterfly—and become it, moving around the underworld like Alice did in Wonderland. I received a lot of good insight from these journeys, but it was during the last dance of the retreat that I had the most freeing shamanic journey, which led me to the upper world instead of the lower world.

The upbeat music and dance began with about fifteen others in the large, dark room where we normally had yoga practice. I was cruising along, shaking my booty and getting into the beat, when I started to gently flap my arms like I was flying softly. I became my spirit animal. I danced and flew gently around for a few songs, and it was peaceful and freeing.

A reggae song came on, and out of nowhere I started moving my arms like I was an animal walking on all fours. Suddenly, I became an all-white baby elephant. I had no idea where this came from, but I went with it and pranced around with one of my arms moving out in front of me like an elephant trunk. This had to look ridiculous to others, but when you have a mask on in total darkness, you can't see anyone else, so you dance like nobody's watching. And by this time in the retreat, everyone had been totally vulnerable, so none of us was judging anyone else.

A new song came on that I don't recall, but when I started to get into it, I became the butterfly again. This time there was a white string tied gently around my midsection, and the other end of the string was tied softly around the neck of a white baby elephant behind me. I began to fly around, and the elephant gracefully followed me wherever I went.

My mind was loving this experience, but it wanted to go

outside the room. I did not physically go outside, but as the white butterfly pulling the elephant, we happily danced outside together in my mind. As the butterfly, I wanted to fly up higher and get a better view of the retreat center. I thought to myself, *I have a four-hundred-pound elephant attached to me. How am I going to get him off the ground?*

As soon as I asked that, I became the elephant again. I was so happy to be guided around by a beautiful butterfly. I could tell that the butterfly wanted to fly, so I just closed my eyes and completely let go of all control. I chose love over fear, and the butterfly gently raised me off the ground until I started to float. We slowly flew up and looked down at the whole retreat center, and there was so much love surrounding it and us.

The butterfly asked me if I wanted to go visit my family in San Diego, and I said yes. We flew across the ocean and hovered over the house. I could see through the roof to my wife, two daughters, and our new puppy all playing together in the living room. I saw a bubble of infinite, unconditional love surrounding each of them. I realized deeply that they were immortal beings and eternally safe inside their bubbles, and that the bubbles would never leave them.

The butterfly started flying up higher and higher, and San Diego became smaller and smaller, until I could see all of California, then all of the United States, including my childhood home in Oklahoma, which was also covered in safe love. The butterfly kept flying, and we flew all the way up into space, where I could see the entire big blue-and-green planet below me.

In space, I became both the butterfly and the elephant at the same time. As both, I just stopped everything and became completely still. I closed my four eyes and just floated in an eternal void of weightless space. I floated there for a few blissful moments in the stillness of Eternal Peace, until I became iridescently clear and dissolved into and became the Eternal Peace.

From this journey, I realized that the present moment is the truest essence of who and what I am, and that for me the butterfly represents the present moment. My body and mind are the elephant. All I have to do is let go completely of trying to control anything or anyone, and choose love over fear, and the present moment will gently and joyfully guide my body and mind for the rest of my days with no effort at all.

My name is Dustin. I am awake, alcohol-free, and complete. The god in me recognizes, honors, and loves the god in you.

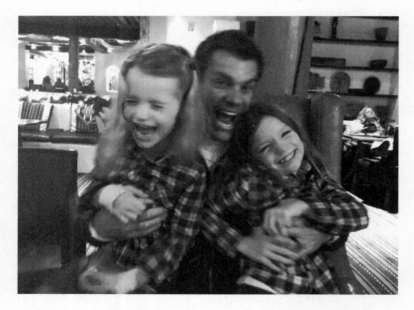

Pure bliss and endless laughter! Celebrating the triumph over alcohol and cherishing the precious moments with my beautiful daughters. Together, we've embraced a brighter, alcohol-free future.

ACKNOWLEDGMENTS

To my daughters:
Do you know what I love about you? Everything! You are the spiritual children of a Universe whose love for you is unconditional and eternal and whose love you are. In every choice in your life, you can either choose to love or fear. There is nothing to fear. Do your absolute best to always choose love.

You are not defective in any way, and you are not the problem when it comes to alcohol. Be extremely careful with alcohol, as it is a cancer-causing, addictive poison that anyone can and will get addicted to once they consume enough. Alcohol suppresses your consciousness. Always remember, you two are Buddhas and could even be the pope one day.

I apologize to the two of you for causing you pain. You have both been so brave and loving to me. You won't consciously remember me when I was addicted, but your unconscious mind will remember, and you will have pain that I caused. I am sorry. I was asleep in the illusion that alcohol benefited me, I didn't realize it was addictive to anyone that consumed enough of it, and

I had unresolved trauma from my childhood. I was unconscious in the alcohol matrix. I am awake now, and the rest of our lives together will be nothing less than magical.

We Dunbars are weird, which is the best compliment there is. When you are weird, it means you are creative and magical. If you ever feel like you're not in a place of peace, joy, or love, just tune back in. Listening in silence is how you can stay in tune. Eternal love is always there for you whenever you need it, and it will never abandon you because you are it at your truest essence.

To the mother of my two beautiful girls:
I am filled with an overwhelming sense of gratitude and admiration for the incredible woman and mother that you are. You have brought immeasurable joy and love into our lives, and your unwavering commitment to our family has touched my heart in ways words can hardly express. Throughout the ups and downs, you have been a pillar of strength and resilience, always putting the needs of our children first. Your nurturing nature, gentle guidance, and endless patience have shaped them into the remarkable individuals they are today. I am in awe of your ability to instill kindness, compassion, and curiosity in their hearts, and I am forever grateful for the loving environment you have created for our family. But beyond your role as a mother, you have also been an incredible friend to me. You have been there to listen, to support, and to share both the joys and the challenges of parenthood. Your unwavering belief in me, even during my moments of doubt, has given me the courage to push forward and be the best father I can be. This book is a testament to the deep bond we share, and it is dedicated not only to our precious daughters but also to you, the woman who has made our journey as parents so incredibly rewarding. Your love, your strength, and your steadfast presence have shaped our lives in

ways that words cannot fully capture. Thank you for being the loving mother our girls deserve and for being the truest friend I could ever ask for. May our story continue to unfold with happiness, love, and countless cherished moments. All my love and gratitude.

To my mom, Linda Dunbar:
This book is a testament to the strength, resilience, and ever-present love that you have shown throughout our family's journey with alcohol addiction. You are a remarkable woman who has endured the pain of witnessing her grandfather, father, husband, and two sons battle this relentless monster. Your continual support and unconditional love have been the pillars that held our family together, providing solace and hope when it seemed all hope was lost. Through this book, I aimed to shed light on the struggles and complexities of alcohol addiction, to unravel its tangled web of emotions, and to offer a glimmer of hope to those who may find themselves entangled in its grip. It is my sincerest wish that this work brings comfort to the hearts of those who have experienced similar journeys and serves as a beacon of understanding for those who have yet to face such trials. Your perseverance in the face of adversity is an inspiration to us all, reminding us that love and compassion can conquer even the darkest of battles. Thank you, Mom, for being the guiding light that leads us toward healing and for showing us the true meaning of love. This book is dedicated to you, with all my love and gratitude.

To my dad, Fred Dunbar (RIP):
I love you and forgive you completely. Your two youngest granddaughters never met you, but they say they would have really liked to. I miss you.

ACKNOWLEDGMENTS

To my Grandma Weezie (RIP):

I am putting up photos of saints, sages, and mystics in my house, and you are going to be right there with them. It is well deserved, Saint Weezie.

To my Grandpa Alva Rose (RIP):

You old buzzard bait, bird dog–smelling, overall-wearing, tobacco-spitting SOB! I am so sorry for the pain and suffering in your life. Your childhood and addictive alcohol caused a ton of misery for you, and that created misery for everyone around you as an adult.

I was so happy to be a part of your life after alcohol. You were every country boy's dream of a grandpa once you overcame your addiction.

To my sister Debi Mahoney:

Your email signature includes the Rumi quote, "Out beyond ideas of wrongdoing and rightdoing, there's a field. I'll meet you there."

Thank you for hanging out with me in that field when I needed you most. For loving me unconditionally. You are a true healer. Your nonjudgmental compassion for others is beyond admirable—it is the goal of life.

To my sister Dayna Dunbar:

You always say you never needed another doll to play with when I came home from the hospital, because I was your real live baby. I know you have always tried your absolute best to make sure I was completely taken care of. Thank you for supporting me so much in everything I do.

To my brother, Darron Dunbar:

You already stole the show, so now what do you want? I know . . . I know . . . some new size eleven, extra-wide silver cowgirl boots that, of course, light up.

You have had a much harder go at life than I have, with many more sacred wound moments. Your continued strength and courage to work through them head-on has been so inspiring to watch from a little brother's view. You have now helped to make the world a better place.

To my father-in-law, Gil Evans: Papa!

I am so sorry for ruining your dinner wine . . . not sorry!

You are the most spiritual man I have ever known, and that is the greatest compliment and the highest gratitude that I can give. For you to show me, not tell me, what true spirituality is has been awe-inspiring to me. Your humbleness is on par with the Dalai Lama, and your never-ending, nonjudgmental support of me even in my darkest hours was pure godliness. Thank you from the bottom of my heart for your unfailing love. I am so happy to call you Dad.

To my mother-in-law, Meg Evans:

OGA (Oh Great Abuela)! You and Gil are the reason your four girls are as strong, beautiful, and successful as they are. Your power shines through them like an eternal beacon.

I know this has been one of the most difficult situations of your life. Your momma bear protection of your daughter has been perfect. You never backed down in my incessant attempt to point my finger elsewhere. Thank you for correctly directing it back at me, for loving me, and . . . for your holiday BBQ turkey! Pure magic.

ACKNOWLEDGMENTS

To Tim Hawks:
Thank you for your constant kindness. You worship my mother, and that means I worship you.

To my good friend Mike Laughlin, AKA my younger brother from another mother: Thank you so much for your unbelievable friendship, generosity, quick wit, humor, and joy. You have all of my gratitude for the year we lived at your house with all of our kids at such a young age. It was one of the happiest times of my life, all because you opened your heart and home to us and helped take care of us like we were your own family. Now we are for sure.

To my dearest friend, Brian Warden:
Growing up next door to one another, you are my longest-tenured brother. Darron is more of a sister, so you get this award.

I have so much gratitude for you always being there for me. Our lives got busy and hectic for a while with kids and work, but all the time I knew you were there when, not if, I needed you.

Boy, did I ever need you, and boy, did you ever come through for me. Thank you so much for our recent trips together, and thank you to your awesome wife, Melissa, for letting you go when I know it was hard on her with all the kids at home and her full-time work. Both you and Melissa's patience and unconditional love for your special needs son, Noah, has been so beautiful to watch, and I have learned so much from you both.

To Andy Earle:
Thank you so much for recording and listening to me ramble on and on and on about alcohol, then, taking it all down and putting it in coherent form. Thank you for all the extra research you did. I am extremely grateful for you.

To my editors, Genet Jones and Miles Doyle:
You are both master wordsmiths! When I handed the manuscript over to you, I thought it was in okay shape. I was beyond wrong. You turned a pile of words into a piece of beautiful art, and I cannot thank you enough.

Most of all, I want to acknowledge and give all of my deepest love and gratitude to the Universe. Thank you for allowing me to be your spiritual offspring, loving me eternally, never abandoning me or judging me, and for the blissful conscious communion with you. The eternal love, patience, and forgiveness that you are is obviously beyond all words. So, I will keep it very simple and say: *thank you, and I love you eternally, too.*

NOTES

INTRODUCTION

1. Kevin D. Shield, Charles Parry, and Jürgen Rehm, "Chronic Diseases and Conditions Related to Alcohol Use," *Alcohol Research: Current Reviews* 35, no. 2 (2014): 155–71, ncbi.nlm.nih.gov/pmc/articles/PMC3908707.

2. Centers for Disease Control and Prevention, "Excessive Alcohol Use Is a Risk to Men's Health," cdc.gov/alcohol/fact-sheets/mens-health.htm.

3. CDC, "Excessive Alcohol Use is a Risk to Men's Health."

4. CDC, "Excessive Alcohol Use is a Risk to Men's Health."

5. CDC, "Excessive Alcohol Use is a Risk to Men's Health."

6. CDC, "Excessive Alcohol Use is a Risk to Men's Health."

7. CDC, "Excessive Alcohol Use is a Risk to Men's Health."

CHAPTER 2

1. RAINN, "Campus Sexual Violence: Statistics," rainn.org/statistics/campus-sexual-violence.

2. Kate B. Carey et al., "Incapacitated and Forcible Rape of College Women: Prevalence across the First Year," *Journal of Adolescent Health* 56, no. 6 (June 2015): 678–80, doi.org/10.1016/j.jadohealth.2015.02.018.

3. Substance Abuse and Mental Health Services Administration, "Facts on College Student Drinking," March 2021, store.samhsa.gov/sites/default/files/pep21-03-10-006.pdf.

4. Gemma Hammerton et al., "Effects of Excessive Alcohol Use on Antisocial Behavior Across Adolescence and Early Adulthood," *Journal of the American Academy of Child & Adolescent Psychiatry* 56, no. 10 (October 2017): 857–65, doi.org/10.1016/j.jaac.2017.07.781.

5. Risë B. Goldstein et al., "The Epidemiology of Antisocial Behavioral Syndromes in Adulthood: Results from the National Epidemiologic Survey on Alcohol and Related Conditions-III," *Journal of Clinical Psychiatry* 78, no. 1 (January 2017): 90–98, doi.org/10.4088/JCP.15m10358.

6. Robert Schlauch, Mathew Waesche, Christina Riccardi, et. al, "A Meta-Analysis of the Effectiveness of Placebo Manipulations in Alcohol-Challenge Studies," *Psychology of Addictive Behaviors* 24, no. 2 (June 2010): 239–53, pubmed.ncbi.nlm.nih.gov/20565150.

CHAPTER 4

1. Lee Benson, "The world's largest and possibly oldest living organism resides in Utah," *Deseret News*, August 15, 2021, deseret.com/utah/2021/8/15/22609608/worlds-largest-and-possibly-oldest-living-organism-resides-in-utah-aspens.

2. "Carl Jung: Analytic Psychology," adapted from Mark Kelland, *Personality Theory in a Cultural Context* (OpenStax CNX, 2015), pdx.pressbooks.pub/

thebalanceofpersonality/chapter/chapter-5-carl-jung/.

3. Quinn Eastman, "Mice Can Inherit Learned Sensitivity to a Smell," Emory News Center, December 2, 2013, news. emory.edu/stories/2013/12/smell_epigenetics_ressler/ campus.html

4. Yasmine Blosse, "From Cool Dudes to Smiley Girls, Males as Predators and Females as Prey: Let's Kick the Stereotypes Out of Kids' Clothing," Action Women, December 11, 2021, actionwomen.org/2021/12/11/from-cool-dudes-to-smiley-girls-males-as-predators-and-females-as-prey-lets-kick-stereotypes-out-of-kids-clothing/.

5. Sam Haysom, "These Charts Show Just How Massive the Gender Divide in Films Really Is," *Mashable*, April 13, 2016, mashable.com/article/film-dialogue-gender-charts.

6. Associated Press, "Americans Are Drinking More Now than When Prohibition Became the Law of the Land," *Los Angeles Times*, January 14, 2020, latimes.com/science/ story/2020-01-14/americans-drinking-more-prohibition.

7. K. Kris Hirst, "History of Alcohol: A Timeline," ThoughtCo, updated May 6, 2019, thoughtco.com/ history-of-alcohol-a-timeline-170889.

8. Patrick E. McGovern, "The Earliest Alcoholic Beverage in the World," Penn Museum, https://www.penn.museum/ research/project.php?pid=12.

9. Amanda Borschel-Dan, "13,000-Year-Old Brewery Discovered in Israel, the Oldest in the World," *The Times of Israel*, September 12, 2018, timesofisrael.com/13000yearoldbrew erydiscoverdinisraeltheoldestintheworld/.

10. Donna Scanlon, "The Whiskey Rebellion," Business Reference Section, Library of Congress, April 2009, loc.gov/

rr/business/businesshistory/August/whiskeyrebellion_rev. html.

11. Pat Strunk, "How Much Does the Average American Drink?" Liquor Laboratory, July 9, 2022, liquorlaboratory. com/how-much-does-the-average-american-drink/.

12. "Prohibition Begins," Business Research Guides, Library of Congress, guides.loc.gov/thismonthinbusinesshistory/ january/prohibition.

CHAPTER 5

1. Robert Ferris, "American Kids See About 3 Alcohol Ads Each Day: Rand Study," CNBC, May 20, 2016, cnbc. com/2016/05/18/american-kids-see-about-3-ads-for-alco hol-each-day-rand-study.html.

2. Sarah Zaske, "Alcohol Ads Can Influence Men and Women to Sexually Coerce Partners," WSU Insider, March 21, 2022, news.wsu.edu/press-release/2022/03/21/alcohol- ads-can-influence-men-and-women-to-sexually-coerce- partners/.

3. Zaske, "Alcohol Ads Can Influence Men and Women to Sexually Coerce Partners."

4. Rebecca L. Collins et al., "Alcohol Advertising Exposure among Middle School–Age Youth: An Assessment across All Media and Venues," *Journal of Studies on Alcohol and Drugs* 77, no. 3 (May 2016): 384–92, doi.org/10.15288/ jsad.2016.77.384.

5. Stuart Elliot, "Liquor Industry Ends Its Ad Ban in Broadcasting," *New York Times*, November 8, 1996, nytimes. com/1996/11/08/business/liquor-industry-ends-its-ad- ban-in-broadcasting.html.

6. Elliot, "Liquor Industry Ends Its Ad Ban in Broadcasting."

7. Dean R. Lillard, Eamon Molly, and Hua Zan, "Television and Magazine Alcohol Advertising: Exposure and Trends by Sex and Age," *Journal of Studies on Alcohol and Drugs* 79, no. 6 (November 2018): 881--92, doi.org/10.15288/jsad.2018.79.881.

8. Lillard, Molly, and Zan, *Journal of Studies on Alcohol and Drugs* 79: 881–92.

9. Lillard, Molly, and Zan, *Journal of Studies on Alcohol and Drugs* 79: 881–92.

10. Lillard, Molly, and Zan, *Journal of Studies on Alcohol and Drugs* 79: 881–92.

11. Lillard, Molly, and Zan, *Journal of Studies on Alcohol and Drugs* 79: 881–92.

12. James Dean, "Exposure to TV Alcohol Ads Linked to Drinking Behavior," *Cornell Chronicle*, May 18, 2020, news.cornell.edu/stories/2020/05/exposure-tv-alcohol-ads-linked-drinking-behavior.

13. Dean, "Exposure to TV Alcohol Ads Linked to Drinking Behavior."

14. Dean, "Exposure to TV Alcohol Ads Linked to Drinking Behavior."

15. Breastcancer.org, "Drinking Alcohol," breastcancer.org/risk/risk-factors/drinking-alcohol.

16. American Cancer Society, "American Cancer Society Guideline for Diet and Physical Activity," cancer.org/healthy/eathealthygetactive/acsguidelinesnutritiophysicalactivitycancerprevention/guidelines.html.

17. Stacy Mosel, "Female Domestic Violence and Alcohol

Use," edited by Kristina Ackerman, reviewed by Ryan Kelley, Alcohol.org, updated March 27, 2023, alcohol.org/women/domestic-abuse-and-alcoholism/.

18. Mosel, "Female Domestic Violence and Alcohol Use."

19. Mosel, "Female Domestic Violence and Alcohol Use."

20. Jef Feeley, "Florida in $879 Million Opioid Settlement With CVS, Allergan and Teva," Bloomberg, March 30, 2022, bloomberg.com/news/articles/2022-03-30/cvs-allergan-teva-to-pay-879-million-in-florida-opioid-accord

CHAPTER 6

1. National Institute on Alcohol Abuse and Alcohoism, "Alcohol Use in the United States: Age Groups and Demographic Characteristics," niaaa.nih.gov/alcoholseffectshealth/alcoholtopics/alcoholfactsandstatistics/alcoholuseunitedstatesagegroupsanddemographiccharacteristics.

2. Nitin Shah, "Operant Conditioning (Punishment and Reward Theory)," Institute of Clinical Hypnosis and Related Sciences, February 26, 2014, instituteofclinicalhypnosis.com/psychotherapy-coaching/operant-conditioning-punishment-and-reward-theory/.

3. Melinda Wenner Moyer, "Hang-xiety? How a Night of Drinking Can Your Mood," *New York Times*, October 6, 2022, nytimes.com/2022/10/06/well/live/hangover-anxiety-mood.html.

4. Nicholas V. Emanuele, Terrence F. Swade, and Mary Ann Emanuele, "Consequences of Alcohol Use in Diabetics," *Alcohol Health and Research World* 22, no. 3 (1998): 211–19, ncbi.nlm.nih.gov/pmc/articles/PMC6761899.

5. Elisa Pabon et al., "Effects of Alcohol on Sleep and

Nocturnal Heart Rate: Relationships to Intoxication and Morning-After Effects," *Alcohol Clinical & Experimental Research* 46, no. 10 (October 2022): 1875–87, doi.org/10.1111/acer.14921.

6. National Center for Complementary and Integrative Health, "Meditation and Mindfulness: What You Need to Know," nccih.nih.gov/health/meditation-and-mindfulness-what-you-need-to-know.

CHAPTER 7

1. Tom Blow, "Jesse Lingard Admits He was 'Drinking to Take the Pain Away' amid Man Utd Struggles," *Daily Mirror*, January 19, 2023, mirror.co.uk/sport/football/news/man-utd-jesse-lingard-forest-28996081.

2. Lamya Khoury et al., "Substance Use, Childhood Traumatic Experience, and Posttraumatic Stress Disorder in an Urban Civilian Population," *Depression and Anxiety* 27, no. 12 (December 2010): 1077–86, doi.org/10.1002/da.20751.

3. Hasan Mirsal et al., "Childhood Trauma in Alcoholics," *Alcohol and Alcoholism* 39, no. 2 (March 2004): 126–29, doi.org/10.1093/alcalc/agh025.

4. Hilary I. Lebow, "Emotional Drinking: Are You Using Alcohol to Feel Better?" reviewed by Alyssa Peckham, Psych Central, updated February 8, 2022, psychcentral.com/addictions/emotional-alcohol-drinking-to-cope.

CHAPTER 8

1. Savage Vines, "The Health Benefits of Organic Wine – Top 5 Reasons," savagevines.co.uk/the-health-benefits-of-organic-wine/.

2. World Health Organization, "Alcohol," May 9, 2022, who. int/news-room/fact-sheets/detail/alcohol.

3. World Health Organization, "Alcohol."

4. World Health Organization, "Alcohol."

5. World Health Organization, "Alcohol."

6. World Health Organization, "Alcohol."

7. International Agency for Research on Cancer, "Agents Classified by the IARC Monographs, Volumes 1–134," updated July 27, 2023, monographs.iarc.who.int/ agents-classified-by-the-iarc/.

8. Cancer Society, "New Cancer Society Campaign Sheds Light on Link between Cancer and Alcohol," May 2022, cancer.org.nz/about-us/cancer-society-media-releases/ new-cancer-society-campaign-sheds-light-on-link-between-cancer-and-alcohol/.

9. Susan Brink, "Alcohol Use Linked to over 740,000 Cancer Cases Last Year, New Study Says," NPR, July 16, 2021, npr. org/sections/goatsandsoda/2021/07/16/1016586837/ new-study-says-nearly-3-4-million-cancers-a-year-linked-to-alcohol-use.

10. Katherine Unger Baillie, "One Alcoholic Drink a Day Linked with Reduced Brain Size," Penn Today, March 4, 2022, penntoday.upenn.edu/news/ one-alcoholic-drink-day-linked-reduced-brain-size.

11. Baillie, "One Alcoholic Drink a Day Linked with Reduced Brain Size."

12. Baillie, "One Alcoholic Drink a Day Linked with Reduced Brain Size."

13. "Alcohol-Related Liver Disease," NHS Inform,

updated May 29, 2023, nhsinform.scot/illnessesand
conditions/stomachliverandgastrointestinaltract/
alcoholrelatedliverdisease.

14. Farah Shirazi, Ashwani K. Singal, and Robert J. Wong,
"Alcohol-Associated Cirrhosis and Alcoholic Hepatitis
Hospitalization Trends in the United States," *Journal
of Clinical Gastroenterology* 55, no. 2 (February 2021):
174–79, doi.org/10.1097/MCG.0000000000001378.

15. "Alcohol-Related Liver Disease," NHS Inform.

16. World Health Organization, "Alcohol."

17. World Health Organization, "Alcohol."

18. Centers for Disease Control and Prevention, "Excessive
Drinking Is Draining the U.S. Economy," reviewed April
14, 2022, cdc.gov/alcohol/features/excessive-drinking.
html.

19. CDC, "Excessive Drinking Is Draining the U.S. Economy."

20. Tapio Paljärvi et al., "Non-employment Histories of
Middle-Aged Men and Women Who Died from
Alcohol-Related Causes: A Longitudinal Retrospec-
tive Study," *PLoS One* 9, no. 5 (May 2014): e98620, doi.
org/10.1371/journal.pone.0098620.

21. Paljärvi et al., *PLoS One* 9: e98620

22. National Coalition for the Homeless, "Substance Abuse
and Homelessness," July 2009, nationalhomeless.org/fact-
sheets/addiction.pdf.

23. National Coalition for the Homeless, "Substance Abuse
and Homelessness."

24. National Coalition for the Homeless, "Substance Abuse
and Homelessness,"

25. Catherine Moore, "Positive Daily Affirmations: Is There Science Behind It?" reviewed by Jo Nash, Positive Psychology, March 4, 2019, positivepsychology.com/daily-affirmations.

CHAPTER 9

1. Robert Williams, "When Dr. Bob Took His Last Drink, Millions Were Saved," *Washington Post*, June 9, 1985, washingtonpost.com/archive/opinions/1985/06/09/when-dr-bob-took-his-last-drink-millions-were-saved/bdd72d91-662e-478d-9a4e-cde9892d6894/.

2. William Silkworth, "Alcoholism as a Manifestation of Allergy," *Medical Record*, March 17, 1937, chestnut.org/resources/8b7ff2b0-522c-4496-8f0a-ede79be1ddc5/1937-Silkworth-Alcoholism-as-Allergy.pdf

3. Silkworth, "Alcoholism as a Manifestation of Allergy," Medical Record.

4. Gabrielle Glaser, "The Irrationality of Alcoholics Anonymous," *The Atlantic*, April 2015, the-atlantic.com/magazine/archive/2015/04/the-irrationality-of-alcoholics-anonymous/386255/.

5. John F. Kelly, Keith Humphreys, and Marica Ferri, " Alcoholics Anonymous and Other 12-Step Programs for Alcohol Use Disorder," *Cochrane Database of Systematic Reviews* 3, no. 3 (Mar 2020): CD012880, doi.org/10.1002/14651858.CD012880.pub2.

6. Chiara Giuliano et al., "Evidence for a Long-Lasting Compulsive Alcohol Seeking Phenotype in Rats," *Neuropsychopharmacology* 43, no. 4 (March 2018): 728–38, doi.org/10.1038/npp.2017.105.

7. The Jackson Laboratory, "Why Are Mice Considered Excellent Models for Humans?" jax.org/why-the-mouse/excellent-models.

8. Annie Grace, *This Naked Mind,* (New York: Avery, 2018), 97.

9. Tenzin Gyatso, "Our Faith in Science," *New York Times,* November 12, 2005, nytimes.com/2005/11/12/opinion/our-faith-in-science.html.

CHAPTER 10

1. Antonio Pierro et al., "'Letting Myself Go Forward past Wrongs': How Regulatory Modes Affect Self-Forgiveness," *PLoS One* 13, no. 3 (March 2018): e0193357, doi.org/10.1371/journal.pone.0193357.

2. Antonio Pierro et al., *PLoS One* 13: e0193357.

3. University of Wisconsin–Madison, "Real Forgiveness Is Never Toxic, Says UW–Madison's Enright to Men's Health," January 10, 2013, education.wisc.edu/news/real-forgiveness-is-never-toxic-says-uw-madisons-enright-to-mens-health/.

4. Man Yee Ho et al., "International REACH Forgiveness Intervention: A Multi-Site Randomized Controlled Trial," OSF Preprints, March 3, 2023, doi.org/10.31219/osf.io/8qzgw.

ABOUT THE AUTHOR

Dustin Dunbar grew up poor in midwestern America with an abusive, alcohol-addicted father and grandfather and vowed to never be like them. Devouring psychology books and researching addiction in his twenties, Dunbar earned a doctorate in psychology and believed at that time that he had broken his family's chains. In 2009, Dunbar was handpicked by Ryan Seacrest for *LA Shrink* and Endemol's *Dallas Life Coach*, where he was the "shrink" and "life coach" on those pilots. After drinking moderately and socially for twenty years, he too became addicted to alcohol. He overcame his addiction at the age of forty-eight and has since been helping others overcome theirs. Dunbar is a coach at WeAretheAFR.org, a nonprofit online community helping others with alcohol addiction and raising consciousness. Dunbar's true passions are spending time with his two young daughters, writing, and sports. He lives in San Diego, California. Learn more at dustin-dunbar.com.